I0816116

Quick Guide to ADHD

Carla Mooney

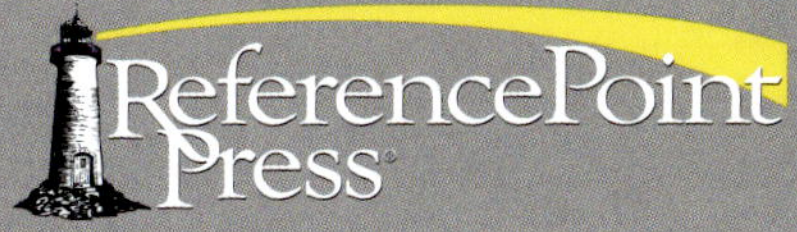

San Diego, CA

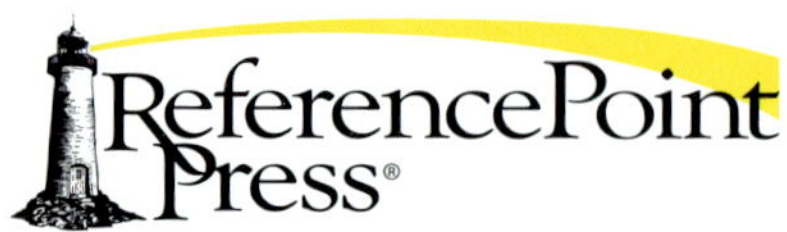

Printed in the United States

For more information, contact:
ReferencePoint Press, Inc.
PO Box 27779
San Diego, CA 92198
www.ReferencePointPress.com

LIBRARY OF CONGRESS CATALOGING-IN-PUBLICATION DATA

Names: Mooney, Carla, 1970- author
Title: Quick guide to ADHD / by Carla Mooney.
Other titles: Quick guide to attention-deficit hyperactivity disorder
Description: San Diego, CA : ReferencePoint Press, Inc, 2026. | Includes bibliographical references and index.
Identifiers: LCCN 2025032657 (print) | LCCN 2025032658 (ebook) | ISBN 9781678212445 library binding | ISBN 9781678212452 ebook
Subjects: LCSH: Attention-deficit hyperactivity disorder--Juvenile literature
Classification: LCC RJ506.H9 M6557 2026 (print) | LCC RJ506.H9 (ebook)
LC record available at https://lccn.loc.gov/2025032657
LC ebook record available at https://lccn.loc.gov/2025032658

CONTENTS

Distracted and Disorganized

When Rohan was in kindergarten, his teachers informed his parents that, although the young boy was very smart, he had trouble paying attention, completing his work, and following directions. Rohan's parents took their son to the doctor, and Rohan was diagnosed with attention-deficit/hyperactivity disorder (ADHD). Rohan's mother, Farah, admits that the ADHD diagnosis stunned her. She worried about how ADHD would impact Rohan's future and whether he would struggle for the rest of his life.

Farah took her son to ADHD specialists at the Children's Hospital of Philadelphia. There clinicians worked with Rohan to find the right medication to manage his ADHD. Over the years, these doctors adjusted Rohan's medication to match his growth stages. Rohan also regularly met with Jenelle Nissley-Tsiopinis, a psychologist in the hospital's Center for Management of ADHD. Nissley-Tsiopinis worked with Rohan to teach him coping and learning strategies.

Like many children with ADHD, Rohan struggled with executive functioning. It was challenging for him to organize his thoughts, manage his time, complete tasks, and make decisions. Often, he got overwhelmed and missed deadlines. Nissley-Tsiopinis worked with Rohan to help him find practical ways to stay organized and succeed in school. "In eighth grade, I was stressed out over homework. She taught me how to break things down and how to organize it. Now I keep track of how long it takes me to do certain types of homework assignments so I can make enough time to get it done, along with other things I like to do. Because I plan, I don't have to rush and get all stressed,"[1] says Rohan, who is now a thirteen-year-old high school freshman.

Every morning, Rohan checks a whiteboard in his room on which he has written down that day's tasks. He carries an accordion binder at school to stay organized in his classes. Because Rohan understands that lack of sleep can make his ADHD symptoms worse, he prioritizes sleep and a regular bedtime so that he is rested for the next day. Rohan has also learned to become his own best advocate and asks for help when he needs it. Sometimes, he will ask a teacher for more explanation on an assignment. At other times, he will discuss an issue with Nissley-Tsiopinis. "He'll tell me, 'I want to work with Dr. Nissley,' so I'll make an appointment," Farah says. "At school, he'll advocate for more time. He has the confidence to do that now. It's exactly what we wanted."[2]

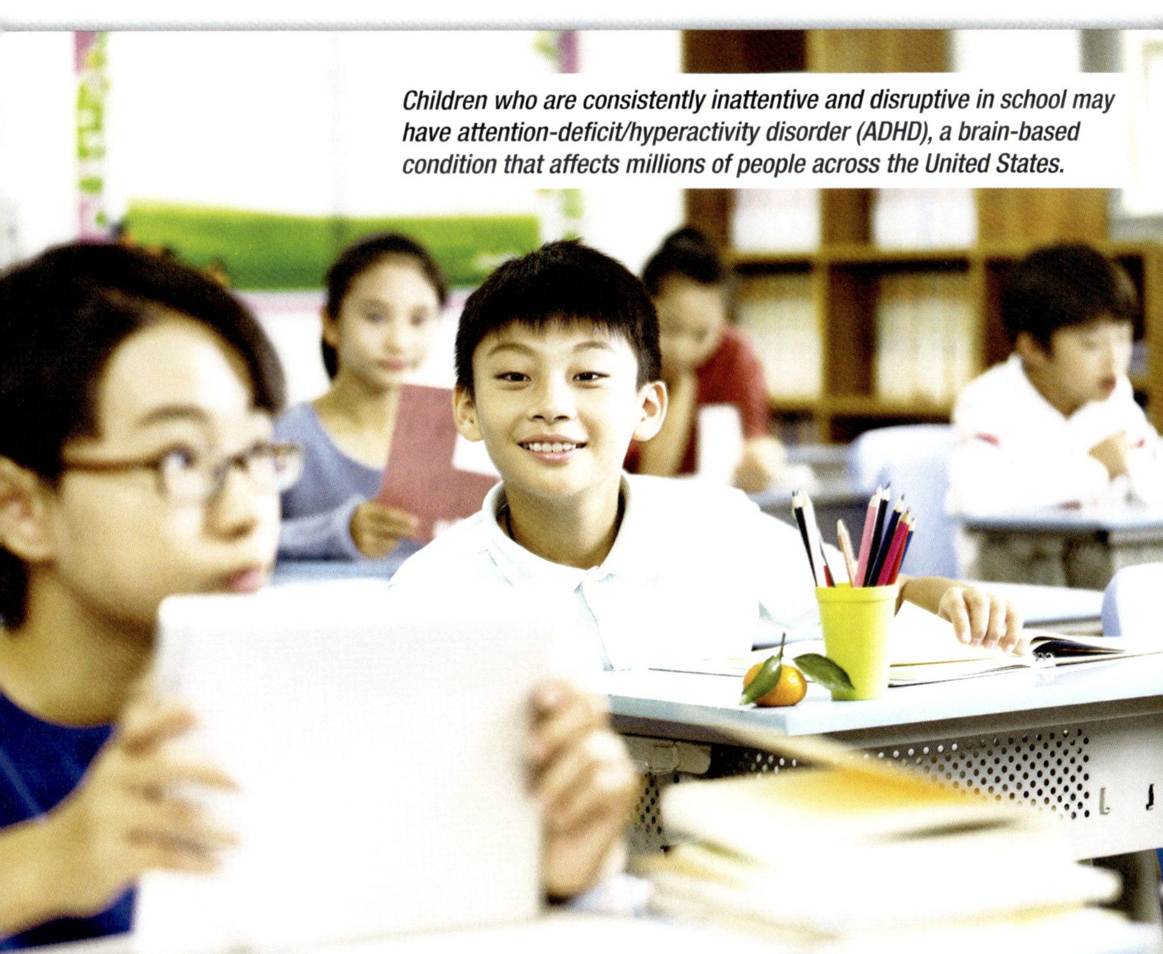

Children who are consistently inattentive and disruptive in school may have attention-deficit/hyperactivity disorder (ADHD), a brain-based condition that affects millions of people across the United States.

Rohan is excited for the future. He is working with Nissley-Tsiopinis to plan out a schedule for SAT preparation. "There's always something to work on for the future and college," Rohan says. "I practice the skills she's taught me. I feel I'm in a great place."[3]

A Brain-Based Disorder

Most people have had trouble paying attention or feeling fidgety at some point in their life. For some individuals, problems with attention, impulsivity, and hyperactivity are persistent and significantly impact their ability to function effectively in school, at work, at home, or in social situations. These people may have ADHD, a common neurodevelopmental disorder. ADHD affects the way the brain functions. People with ADHD often have trouble focusing, staying still, and controlling their actions. ADHD symptoms typically begin in childhood but can affect people of all ages.

ADHD impacts millions of people across the United States. Approximately 7 million US children aged three to seventeen (11.4 percent of the population) had been diagnosed with ADHD as of 2022, according to the Centers for Disease Control and Prevention (CDC). An estimated 15.5 million US adults had also been diagnosed with ADHD as of 2023, according to the CDC. About half of those adults did not receive a diagnosis until they were adults. Experts believe that many more people have ADHD but have not been officially diagnosed.

> **"We all know people with ADHD who have learned to cope with it, found their niche, and are doing very well. That is one of the most promising things about ADHD."[4]**
>
> **—Andrea Chronis-Tuscano, psychology professor at the University of Maryland**

Although there is no cure for ADHD, treatments such as medication, therapy, and lifestyle changes can help manage symptoms. "We all know people with ADHD who have learned to cope with it, found their niche, and are doing very well. That is one of the most promising things about ADHD,"[4] says Andrea Chronis-Tuscano, a psychology professor at the University of Maryland who specializes in ADHD. This common disorder can be managed and does not stop individuals from performing at their best.

CHAPTER ONE

ADHD: A Brain-Based Condition

Denise Moss was concerned about her son, Kyle. In grade school, Kyle had trouble paying attention and struggled to finish tasks. He was always on the move and never able to sit still. Moss decided to take Kyle to a doctor, who diagnosed him with ADHD. Later, her younger son, Blake, was also diagnosed with ADHD. Moss wanted to learn more about the disorder to help her children, and she signed up for a presentation about ADHD.

At one point in the presentation, the speaker explained how ADHD can appear differently in women. For Moss, it was as if the speaker was describing her life. For years, Moss had struggled to finish tasks at home, lost keys, and was generally unorganized. She often wondered why everyday activities were so difficult for her and worried that it made her a bad mother and wife. Now she had a potential answer for her symptoms: ADHD.

Moss consulted with a psychiatric nurse practitioner and was diagnosed with ADHD. She and her sons, who are now twelve and fourteen years old, started medication to help control their ADHD symptoms. She believes that her diagnosis has helped her transform her life and made her a better mother. She has created a daily routine and structure, including keeping a detailed calendar and using colored sticky notes to remind herself and the boys of tasks that must be completed. Now all three are thriving.

Learning how to manage her ADHD has also improved Moss's self-image. "I always felt dumb," she says. "But it was because I couldn't give my best effort."[5]

Differences in the Brain

Over the years, scientists have studied the brains of people with and without ADHD in detail. They use structural imaging such as computed tomography scans and magnetic resonance imaging to create two- and three-dimensional images of the brain. These images reveal structural differences in the brains of individuals with ADHD, particularly in areas that play a crucial role in focus and attention.

Brain imaging studies reveal that children with ADHD often have a smaller prefrontal cortex than children without the disorder. This area of the brain is highly involved in executive functioning. Individuals use executive function skills to manage daily tasks, including setting goals, staying organized, managing time, and completing tasks. Also, the prefrontal cortex in a child with ADHD matures more slowly compared to that of children without the disorder. The structural difference in the prefrontal cortex may be a factor in many of the symptoms of ADHD, which involve problems with executive function skills.

"I always felt dumb. But it was because I couldn't give my best effort."[5]

—Denise Moss, adult diagnosed with ADHD

Other brain areas—such as the cerebellum, hippocampus, and amygdala—are also often smaller in children with ADHD. The cerebellum is involved in the ability to suppress actions that interrupt a current task, such as staying seated during class. The hippocampus and amygdala play crucial roles in regulating memory, emotion, and behavior. The smaller size may disrupt these functions, leading to some of the symptoms experienced by children with ADHD.

As a child grows and matures, their brain changes. The structural differences observed in the brains of children with ADHD may persist into adulthood. Researchers following adolescents

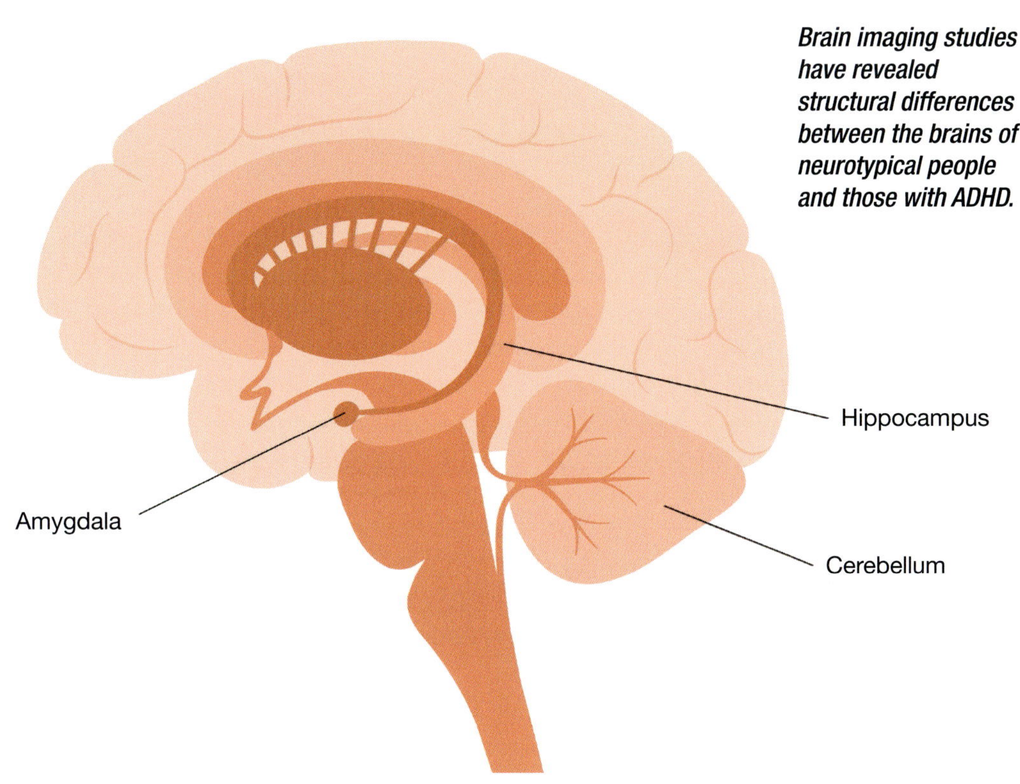

Brain imaging studies have revealed structural differences between the brains of neurotypical people and those with ADHD.

diagnosed with ADHD at age sixteen into adulthood found that they still had smaller brain volume as adults and poorer memory function compared to adults without ADHD. In particular, the caudate nucleus, a brain region that coordinates information across different parts of the brain and supports cognitive and memory functions, was found to be smaller in volume in the brains of individuals with ADHD. Since the brain's structural differences remain in adulthood for most people with ADHD, researchers believe that most people diagnosed with ADHD as children will continue to experience many of its symptoms as adults.

Neural Networks and Connectivity

Scientists have also investigated how different brain regions communicate with each other in individuals with ADHD. Brain cells called neurons work together in a neural network to send messages from one part of the brain to another. The brain uses its neural networks to process information, send motor commands,

A Brief History of ADHD

Although the term *ADHD* has only been around for a few decades, medical practitioners have noticed its symptoms for centuries. In 1798 Alexander Crichton, a Scottish physician, noted that certain individuals under his care could not consistently focus on tasks, and in the early 1900s, doctors identified children who exhibited impulsive, uncontrolled behaviors despite being quite intelligent. Over time, medical authorities used different terms to describe the condition, such as minimal brain dysfunction or hyperkinetic reaction of childhood.

In the 1980s doctors started to use *attention deficit disorder* to categorize this behavior. Recognizing that some people with attention issues also had problems with hyperactivity and impulsiveness, the American Psychiatric Association's *Diagnostic and Statistical Manual of Mental Disorders* renamed the condition attention-deficit/hyperactivity disorder (ADHD) in 1987.

Though it has been observed for centuries, ADHD is still often undiagnosed. Children with ADHD are often dismissed as lazy, undisciplined, or the result of bad parenting. Some people believe children with ADHD will eventually grow out of it. However, proper medical diagnosis recognizes ADHD as a condition that affects how the brain develops and functions. Understanding this helps guide effective treatment and support for those with ADHD.

and perform cognitive functions, including those related to learning and memory. Signals travel through the brain's neural network through different pathways and areas of the brain depending on the messages being sent and the type of information being processed.

Scientists have identified differences in how the brain's neural networks function in people with ADHD. Functional magnetic resonance imaging (fMRI) measures blood flow in the brain, which is an indicator of brain activity. In active areas of the brain, blood flow increases. Using fMRI scans, scientists have discovered that people with ADHD have different patterns of activity in areas of the brain linked to cognitive, emotional, and motor regulation. These differences may explain some of the characteristics of ADHD, such as impulsivity, hyperactivity, and trouble with attention and focus.

One area believed to be involved in ADHD is the anterior cingulate cortex, a region of the brain that plays a significant role in attention. The anterior cingulate cortex is involved in adjusting the focus of a person's attention and balancing how much attention is used and for how long. Studies of people with and without ADHD as they performed a challenging cognitive task revealed a difference in how the brain responded. While the non-ADHD group activated their anterior cingulate cortex during the task, the ADHD group did not. Instead, the ADHD group used a different part of the brain during the task. These results suggest that the ADHD group's inability to activate the anterior cingulate cortex, the most effective part of the brain for attention, made it more difficult to focus on the challenging task.

Another brain area believed to be involved in ADHD is the default mode network (DMN). The DMN is a connected group of brain areas that is usually most active when the brain is at rest or daydreaming. When a person engages in a task, the DMN's activity typically decreases, allowing other brain areas to increase their activity and focus attention on the task. However, in children with ADHD, the DMN does not slow down when the attention and cognitive control networks fire up. The DMN remains unusually active when these children attempt to concentrate on a task. Some research suggests that weak connections between the DMN and cognitive control networks are responsible for this disconnect. This difference may be part of the reason why children with ADHD struggle to focus and pay attention.

A 2024 study from researchers at the National Institutes of Health has also linked symptoms of ADHD with unusual connections between the brain's frontal cortex and information processing centers deep in the brain. The researchers reviewed thousands of functional brain images from people with and without ADHD. They found that youth with ADHD had increased brain activity connecting deep brain structures involved in learning, movement, reward, and emotion with structures in the frontal cortex involved in attention and control of unwanted behaviors. "The findings from this study help further our understanding of the brain processes contributing to ADHD symptoms. Such understanding is a first step in thinking of new ways to help those

> "Brain changes are only part of the story. ADHD is a complex condition, and many other changes in brain connectivity will play a role."[6]
>
> —Philip Shaw, researcher at the National Institutes of Health

who find the symptoms cause difficulties in day-to-day life," says Philip Shaw, one of the study's leaders. "But these brain changes are only part of the story. ADHD is a complex condition, and many other changes in brain connectivity will play a role."[6]

Neurotransmitter Activity

Chemical imbalances in the brain may also be a factor in ADHD symptoms. Brain chemicals called neurotransmitters help the brain send messages from one brain region to another. One important neurotransmitter is dopamine. Dopamine has several roles in the brain related to motivation, attention, and reward. Studies suggest that people with ADHD may have lower levels of dopamine or problems with how dopamine is used in the brain.

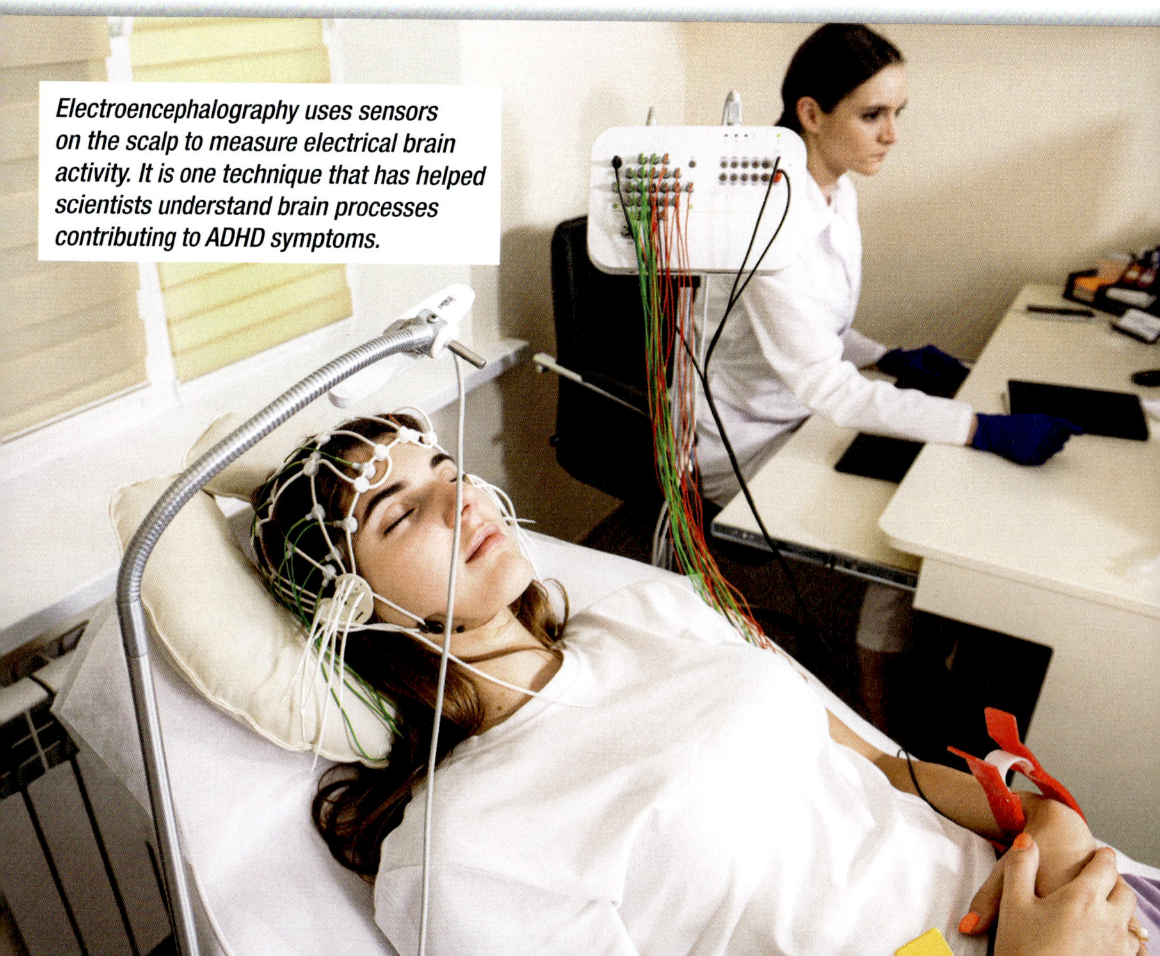

Electroencephalography uses sensors on the scalp to measure electrical brain activity. It is one technique that has helped scientists understand brain processes contributing to ADHD symptoms.

Types of ADHD

Doctors divide ADHD into three categories based on specific symptoms. People with "ADHD predominantly inattentive presentation" mainly struggle with focus and attention to tasks. They might be forgetful, disorganized, and easily distracted but not overly active or impulsive. Predominantly inattentive presentation is more common in young girls and may go unnoticed until school demands increase. Often labeled as shy, quiet, or even unmotivated, these students are usually working hard to keep up.

People with "ADHD predominantly hyperactive–impulsive presentation" typically have symptoms of hyperactivity and impulsivity but not inattention. They may talk constantly, interrupt others, or struggle with self-control. Predominantly hyperactive–impulsive presentation is more common in young children, especially boys. These children often get in trouble at school for behavior that others see as disruptive, even though they may be bright and eager to learn.

The most common form of ADHD is "ADHD combined presentation." People with this form of ADHD have a mix of inattention, hyperactivity, and impulsivity symptoms. The symptoms may shift over time, and different traits may stand out in different settings. For example, a child might be very hyper at home but mostly inattentive at school. This mix can complicate diagnosis, since symptoms do not always follow a clear pattern.

These differences can make it harder for them to stay interested in tasks, control their behavior, or feel motivated.

Although scientists have identified differences in the structure, function, and chemistry of the brains of people with ADHD, they still do not fully understand how these differences cause ADHD symptoms. Not everyone with ADHD has the same brain differences or symptoms.

ADHD and Executive Function

ADHD can have a significant impact on a person's executive function skills. Executive function skills are a set of mental skills that enable a person to plan, focus attention, remember instructions, and manage multiple tasks effectively. These skills are like the brain's management system.

People with ADHD often struggle with executive functions. For example, they may struggle to initiate tasks or maintain focus, overlook steps in a task or miss details, become easily distracted, or have difficulty organizing materials or managing their time. They may also act impulsively without thinking through the consequences, or struggle to regulate their emotions.

Imagine trying to bake a cake but forgetting to preheat the oven, skipping important ingredients, or walking away in the middle of baking. That is what everyday life can feel like for someone with ADHD. These challenges do not arise because a person is lazy or careless. They occur because there are real differences in how the ADHD brain processes and manages information.

What Causes ADHD?

Scientists believe that ADHD does not have a single cause. Instead, they suspect ADHD results from a combination of genetic and environmental factors that affect brain development. One significant risk factor for ADHD is genetics. "There are many contributing factors or risk factors that can contribute to ADHD, but we know the biggest player looks to be more genetics,"[7] says pediatrician Jonathan Shook. If a parent or close relative has ADHD, there is a higher chance that the child will also have it. Studies of families and twins show that ADHD often runs in families.

> **"There are many contributing factors or risk factors that can contribute to ADHD, but we know the biggest player looks to be more genetics."[7]**
>
> —Jonathan Shook, pediatrician

Scientists are investigating many genes that may play a role in ADHD. Some of these genes are linked to the neurotransmitter dopamine. However, researchers believe that no single gene causes ADHD. Instead, they believe a combination of many genes increases a person's risk of developing ADHD. "We don't know of one specific gene, but it's more polygenetic, which means there are lots of genetic regions that are being looked at,"[8] says Shook.

Along with genes, environmental factors can also increase a person's risk of developing ADHD. These may affect a person's developing brain before or shortly after birth, causing the cerebral changes observed in ADHD. Some environmental factors that have been linked to ADHD include exposure to lead or pesticides

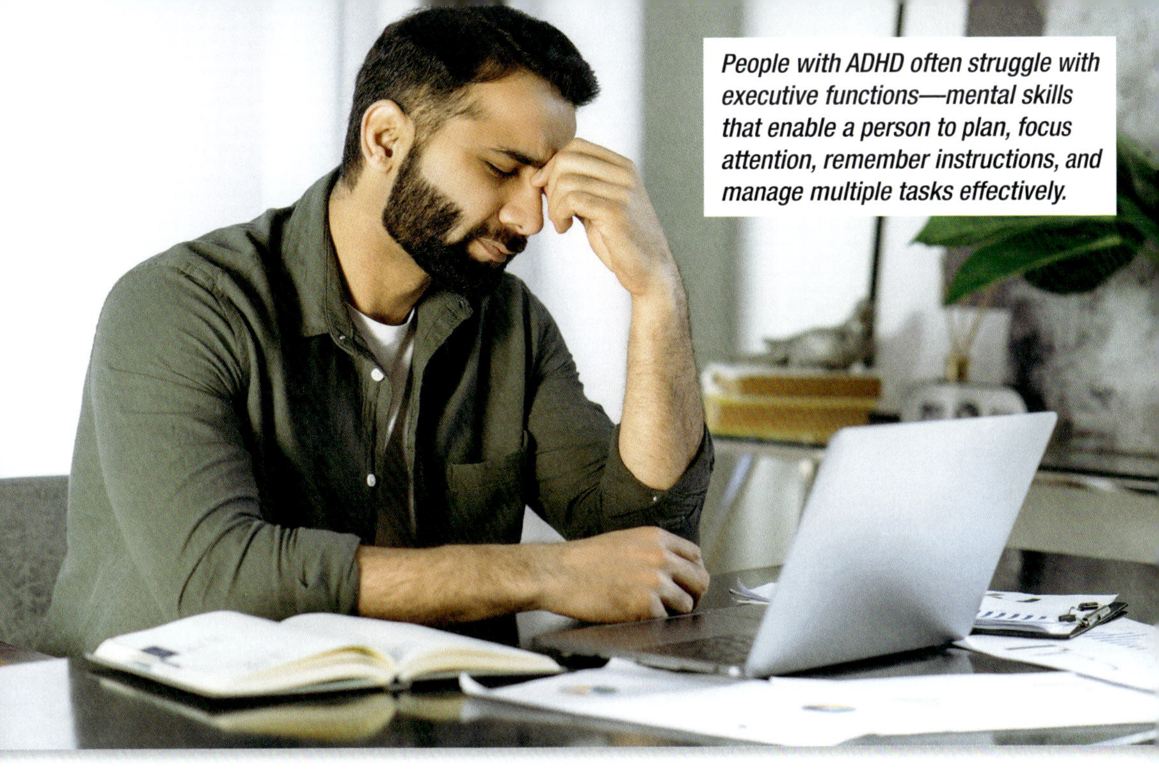

People with ADHD often struggle with executive functions—mental skills that enable a person to plan, focus attention, remember instructions, and manage multiple tasks effectively.

in early childhood; premature birth or low birth weight; exposure to alcohol, cigarette smoke, or drugs while in the uterus; and a serious brain injury. However, more research is needed to understand how these factors interact with genetics to affect brain development. "Children who have an underlying tendency for ADHD or have that trait or genes, we know that going through certain environments or stressors are more likely to cause symptoms to be noticeable or come out,"[9] Shook says.

A Complex Condition

ADHD is a complex neurological condition. Understanding the unique ways that the brain works in people with ADHD helps explain why people with the disorder face challenges in attention, self-control, and organization. Scientists continue to study how the brain develops and how genetics and environmental influences contribute to ADHD. By learning how ADHD impacts impulse control and concentration, scientists and medical experts can better determine what can be done to support people with the disorder throughout their lives.

CHAPTER TWO

Symptoms and Diagnosis

Diagnosed with ADHD as a child, Sophie Knight displayed many classic ADHD symptoms. In school and at home, she often struggled to focus her attention and had trouble sitting still. In fact, Knight's near-constant movement led her family to call her "Tigger" after the bouncy tiger from the well-known Winnie-the-Pooh stories. At the same time, Knight could be hyper-focused on tasks she enjoyed, such as reading a book.

As an adult, Knight still experiences ADHD symptoms. Her mind often gets distracted by a stream of changing thoughts. Even sitting down to watch an hour of television can be a challenge. "I'll get up maybe five times, because my brain tells me I need to fetch lip balm, get tea, take off my nail polish, text five people, stretch, do the washing-up, organize my desk," she says. And once she starts something, finishing it can be another challenge. "I can set a pan on the stove, turn it on, and think, 'I'll just get the cushions off the balcony before it rains,' but then I'll start watering the plants, and before I know it, the kitchen is full of smoke,"[10] Knight says.

Knight describes what living with ADHD feels like, saying, "Untamed ADHD feels, to me, like I have a fire hose of information spraying at me all the time. It feels like those game shows where they put cash in wind machines and you're trying to grab the notes, but you just can't. So I'll be at a meeting and it feels like this torrent of information is rushing past me, and I'm just missing whole chunks of it."[11]

Signs and Symptoms

ADHD looks different in everyone. Some may be constantly moving and full of energy, while others seem quiet but cannot stay focused. ADHD symptoms typically fall into three main categories: inattention, hyperactivity, and impulsiveness. A person with ADHD may show signs from any combination of these categories. Symptoms can also range from mild to severe and can change over time.

> **"Untamed ADHD feels, to me, like I have a fire hose of information spraying at me all the time. It feels like those game shows where they put cash in wind machines and you're trying to grab the notes, but you just can't."[11]**
>
> **—Sophie Knight, adult living with ADHD**

Many people with ADHD experience hyperactivity. They might feel restless or need to move constantly. They might fidget, squirm, and have trouble staying seated. Children with hyperactivity might climb or run when they are not supposed to and struggle to participate in quiet activities. In social situations, a person may talk excessively or interrupt others. ADHD's hyperactivity symptoms are often more noticeable in younger children and lessen as they grow older. In teens and adults, hyperactivity may appear as feeling restless, having trouble relaxing, or experiencing an urge to stay busy.

Olivia Chavez often got into trouble as a child because of her hyperactive ADHD symptoms. She says:

> The hyperactivity really felt like I just had to get up and move. And it was very easy when I was playing outside with my sister and we had a group of kids in the neighborhood where my grandma lived where we would all run around. So there was no issue there. Really, where I noticed it was during school, once I had to be disciplined and listening, or in church as well. That was the most difficult because I felt like I had to get up and move and run around. Or sometimes [it] would even manifest itself in needing to talk, just any sort of movement in my body. And it was really hard to repress that.[12]

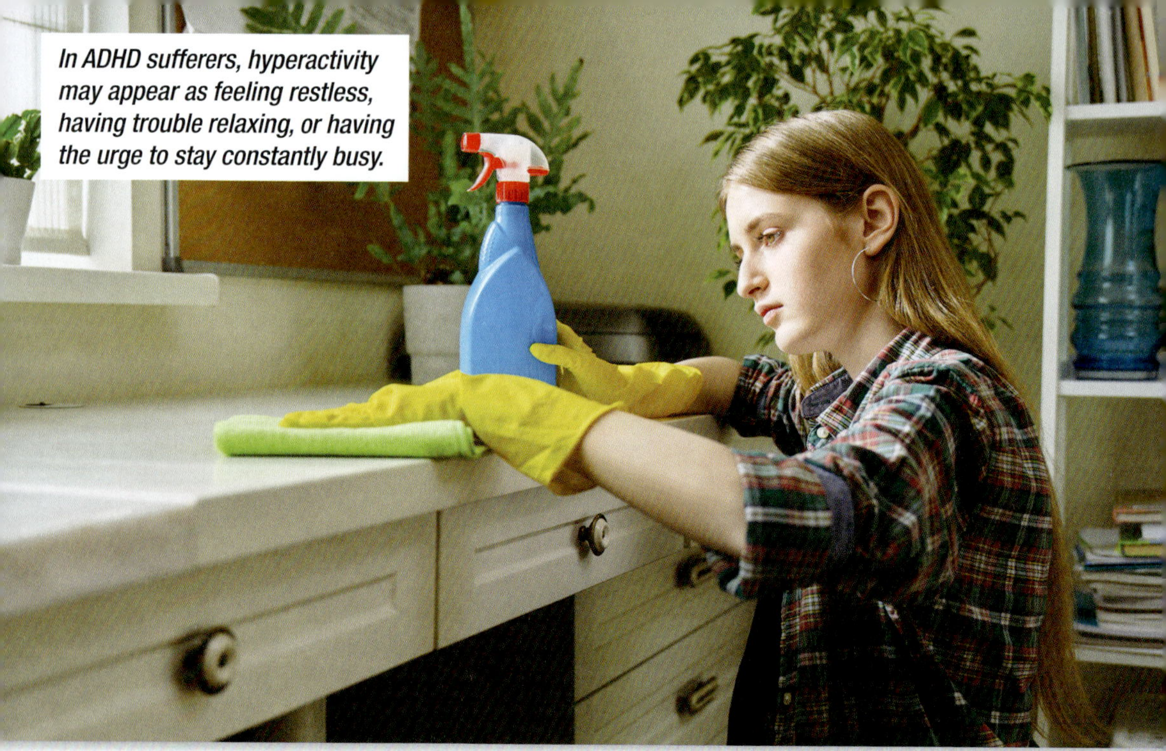

In ADHD sufferers, hyperactivity may appear as feeling restless, having trouble relaxing, or having the urge to stay constantly busy.

ADHD can also cause impulsive behavior. People might act before thinking, interrupt conversations, shout out answers in class, and have trouble waiting their turn. Sometimes, impulsiveness can lead people to take risks without considering the consequences. Impulsive behavior can make it harder for people to make friends or succeed in school because they may appear rude or get into trouble for not following classroom rules.

The ADHD symptom of inattentiveness can be more challenging to recognize because it often does not involve loud, visible behaviors. Instead, a student may stare out the window during class or forget instructions for a class assignment. Such individuals have trouble staying focused, struggle with organization, and get easily distracted. They frequently forget things, misplace items, and fail to meet deadlines. They make careless mistakes in assignments.

ADHD in Girls

For a long time, people believed that ADHD mainly affected boys. Boys with ADHD often display visible symptoms, including hyperactivity and impulsiveness. At school, they might run around the classroom or talk disruptively. Girls with ADHD, especially those with the inattentive type of ADHD, may be more likely to daydream, feel anxious, or struggle quietly. They are also more likely than boys to try to cover up their symptoms and fit in, even if they feel different.

> **"Symptoms of ADHD in girls and women can be more subtle and harder to recognize. That can delay diagnosis."[13]**
>
> —Lisa MacLean, psychiatrist at Henry Ford Health

Because of these differences, girls are often diagnosed later than boys and sometimes not at all. Teachers and parents might think a girl is just shy or forgetful and not realize she has ADHD. Even when a girl shows signs of hyperactivity or impulsiveness, adults may still not recognize it as signs of ADHD. As a result, boys are three times more likely to be diagnosed with ADHD than girls, according to the CDC. "That doesn't necessarily mean that fewer girls have ADHD. But symptoms of ADHD in girls and women can be more subtle and harder to recognize. That can delay diagnosis,"[13] says Lisa MacLean, a psychiatrist at Henry Ford Health in Michigan.

MacLean explains that girls with ADHD are more likely to have inattentive behaviors. They may be easily distracted or forgetful and have trouble following directions. Their inattention to detail can lead to careless mistakes and difficulty staying organized and on task. In girls, hyperactivity and impulsiveness may be more subtle and appear as fidgeting, racing thoughts, or speaking out before thinking.

ADHD as Part of a Behavioral Continuum

ADHD is often assessed by looking at a range of behaviors or struggles across people's lives. This means that the symptoms associated with ADHD—such as inattention, hyperactivity, and impulsiveness—can appear in all people to varying degrees. Some individuals may experience these traits more intensely or more frequently, which can interfere with daily life and lead to an ADHD diagnosis. Others may show milder symptoms that do not meet the full criteria for an ADHD diagnosis but still cause challenges. Understanding ADHD as a part of a continuum of occasionally disruptive behaviors or lack of mental focus highlights that everyone's experience with ADHD is different. While one person may struggle mostly with attentiveness, another may find it harder to manage emotions or stay organized. Assessing ADHD symptoms in relation to a broader range of behavioral patterns and mental processes allows educators, doctors, and families to provide personalized support based on individual needs rather than adopting a one-size-fits-all approach.

"Girls (and women) are more likely to have inattentive behaviors. But that doesn't mean that's their only symptom," says MacLean. Girls with ADHD hyperactive symptoms often act differently than boys with the same symptoms. "Unlike the stereotypical presentation of a boy who's jumping up and down and getting in classmates' faces, girls with ADHD may just seem energetic, talkative and social. Since girls often display fewer behavioral problems and less noticeable symptoms, their difficulties are often overlooked,"[14] she says. Because their symptoms are harder to recognize, girls are less likely than boys to be evaluated and treated for ADHD.

ADHD in Adults

ADHD is not just a childhood condition. Many children and teens with ADHD experience symptoms into adulthood, although their symptoms often change over time. For some, hyperactivity becomes less noticeable; however, problems with focus, organization, and impulsive behavior can persist.

Sometimes, those who live with ADHD are not diagnosed until they are adults. In fact, many adults with ADHD do not realize they have the disorder unless diagnosed. For some, seeing their child's ADHD struggles and diagnosis causes them to recognize the signs of ADHD in their own lives.

Adults with ADHD most commonly have symptoms of inattention, impulsiveness, and restlessness. Symptoms vary from person to person and can range from mild to severe. Many adults with ADHD have trouble focusing and prioritizing tasks. They struggle with time management and meeting deadlines. They may have difficulty planning and organizing, which can lead to missing appointments, forgetting social plans, and losing items. They might interrupt others during conversations, grow impatient waiting in line, and experience mood swings and angry outbursts.

For most of her life, Terry Matlen, a clinical social worker, felt that something was just "off." As a child, she struggled with anxiety and had trouble paying attention in class and staying organized. Yet no one recognized that she had ADHD. The challenges

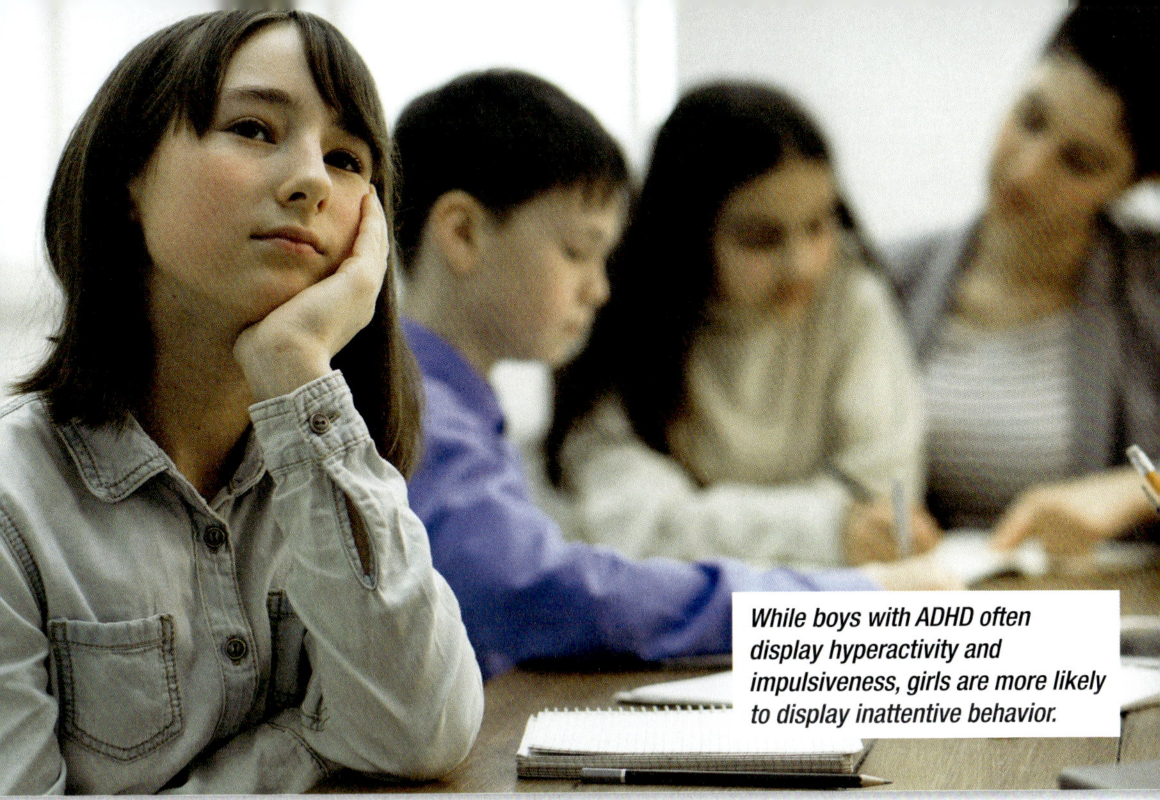

While boys with ADHD often display hyperactivity and impulsiveness, girls are more likely to display inattentive behavior.

followed Matlen into adulthood. It was not until she was in her forties and her daughter was diagnosed with ADHD that Matlen realized that she, too, might have the disorder. After consulting with her doctor, Matlen was diagnosed with ADHD. "This makes sense now. I can't concentrate; I can't finish projects; my house is a disaster; I can't get dinner on the table," Matlen says. "Anxiety doesn't explain the extent of my disorganization." Receiving a diagnosis gave Matlen a sense of relief; she finally had an explanation for how she felt her whole life. Part of her, however, wishes that she had been diagnosed earlier. "There is a lot of grief work that needs to be done to help work through the many years of struggling and not knowing why,"[15] Matlen says.

Diagnosing ADHD: What to Expect

There is no single test to diagnose ADHD. Instead, diagnosis is a process with several steps that involve gathering information and ruling out other causes of symptoms. Often, the path to diagnosis begins at home or school. Parents, teachers, or the individuals themselves may notice signs of ADHD that interfere with daily activities, including patterns of inattention, hyperactivity, or impulsivity that are more intense than what is usual for others of the same age. These symptoms typically appear before age twelve and must be observed in more than one setting, such as both at home and at school.

Trained health professionals—such as doctors, psychologists, or psychiatrists—conduct ADHD screenings. As part of a screening, one of these clinicians will review a patient's behavior at home, school, or work. Often, the clinician will ask parents, teachers, and other caregivers to complete questionnaires about a person's behavior as part of the screening. The clinician will also gather information about a person's medical history and development to rule out other conditions that may cause similar symptoms, such as sleep disorders or mental health disorders. Then the focus will shift to a person's symptoms, how long they have been occurring, how frequently they occur, and what, if any, problems they cause in the person's life. A doctor will also perform a physical examination to rule out any underlying medical issues, such as vision or hearing problems, thyroid disorders, or nutritional deficiencies.

Health care professionals follow guidance in the fifth edition of the American Psychiatric Association's *Diagnostic and Statistical Manual of Mental Disorders* (DSM-5) to help diagnose ADHD in patients. For an ADHD diagnosis, children up to age sixteen must display six or more symptoms combined of inattention or

Coexisting Conditions

Many people with ADHD also have coexisting conditions. Common coexisting conditions include learning disorders such as dyslexia or problems with math, mood disorders such as depression or bipolar disorder, anxiety disorders, tics and Tourette's syndrome, sleep disorders, autism spectrum disorder, and disruptive behavior disorders. In fact, more than two-thirds of individuals with ADHD have at least one other diagnosis. Coexisting conditions often share symptoms with ADHD, which can make diagnosis and treatment more complicated. Additionally, coexisting conditions can make ADHD symptoms more severe. In many cases, when a person has ADHD and another diagnosed condition, doctors may choose to confront ADHD symptoms first because the treatment may reduce stress, improve attention, and increase a person's ability to handle symptoms from the coexisting condition.

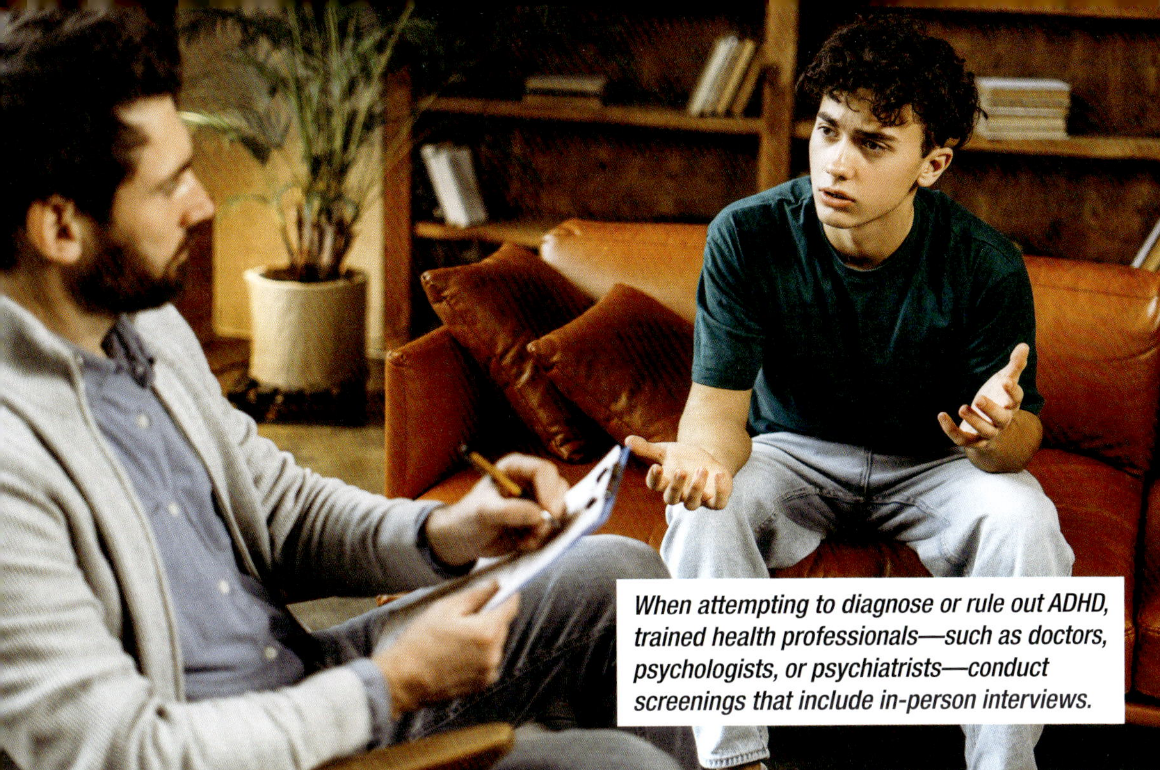

When attempting to diagnose or rule out ADHD, trained health professionals—such as doctors, psychologists, or psychiatrists—conduct screenings that include in-person interviews.

hyperactivity–impulsivity as described in the DSM-5. People aged seventeen and older must display five or more symptoms of inattention or hyperactivity–impulsivity.

Why Diagnosis Matters

For many people, getting an ADHD diagnosis is a relief. Receiving a diagnosis helps patients understand why they struggle and provides them with a path forward. Without a diagnosis, individuals with ADHD might be misunderstood as lazy, defiant, or unmotivated. They may suffer from low self-esteem and feel like they can never succeed. Finding an explanation for their challenges can help people feel better about themselves. Thirty-two-year-old Kelly was able to let go of her self-doubt and negative feelings after her ADHD diagnosis. She says:

> The validation and relief I felt holding the paperwork with the ADHD diagnosis in my hand was the most pivotal moment in my adult life to this day. For the first time in my life, I felt

> seen and understood, and I felt I could finally see myself and give myself the compassion I deserved. After years of lost friendships, missed deadlines, late arrivals, breakdowns, depression, and anxiety I had come to believe I was unmotivated, emotional, strange, annoying, clueless, and selfish. When I was diagnosed with ADHD, these beliefs I had about myself changed. I began to view myself with compassion. I realized that coming up short so much of my life wasn't a moral failure—it was a difference in the structures and chemistry in my brain.[16]

The earlier that patients are diagnosed with ADHD, the earlier that they can get the support they need and develop strategies to manage their symptoms, including receiving accommodations at school, visiting a therapist, and learning coping skills. With the right help, people with ADHD thrive in school, work, and life. "ADHD is a real medical condition that shows up differently in patients—often depending on whether they are adults or children, and whether they are male or female," says Shanta Whitaker, managing director of Continuum Health Group, a Washington, DC, public health and health disparities policy firm. "With millions of American children and adults diagnosed with ADHD, we must work together to be sure that patients get the right type of diagnosis and care."[17]

CHAPTER THREE

Treatment Options

Sixteen-year-old Rory Manson was diagnosed with ADHD in the fourth grade. Rory was a good student, but she often daydreamed in class and frequently forgot to bring her textbooks and schoolwork home. Homework assignments were not hard for Rory, but sitting down to finish them was a challenge. At age nine, Rory began taking ADHD medication to help her manage her symptoms. Medication made Rory's symptoms improve for several years, but by the seventh grade, Rory was struggling under a more intense workload at school.

To help get back on track, Rory began weekly meetings via phone and email with Jodi Sleeper-Triplett, an ADHD coach in Virginia. During these conversations, Rory shared her challenges and successes with her coach. Sleeper-Triplett says:

> [Rory's] full of ideas and really wants to succeed. The problem was that Rory lacked the basic skills needed for success. At first, our discussions focused on organization, although we also spent a lot of time exploring why it was such a struggle for her to reach her goals. Why did it take her so long to get ready for school each morning? Why did she have so much trouble finishing her homework? The answer was always the same: procrastination.[18]

Sleeper-Triplett helped Rory learn skills that she could use in school and at home to manage her time and provide the daily structure she needed in order to succeed. At home,

> **"Distractibility was a problem for Rory at school as well as at home. The moment she felt bored by the material being covered in class, she'd turn to a friend and strike up a conversation. She realized that she needed to separate herself physically from her friends so she wouldn't do this."[19]**
>
> **—Jodi Sleeper-Triplett, ADHD coach**

Rory scheduled time to clean her room, pack her backpack, and organize for the next day. She began doing homework in the kitchen and put her cell phone away until she finished to minimize distractions. If she did not have homework in a class, Rory spent twenty minutes reviewing class material, which helped her meet her academic goals. Sleeper-Triplett says:

> Distractibility was a problem for Rory at school as well as at home. The moment she felt bored by the material being covered in class, she'd turn to a friend and strike up a conversation. She realized that she needed to separate herself physically from her friends so she wouldn't do this. When she talks to her friends in *between* classes, she's careful to include schoolwork in the conversation. That helps her remember her assignments.[19]

Rory's ADHD no longer holds her back. She is performing well in school and plans to attend college after graduation. Many young people like Rory with ADHD experience major improvements in their daily lives when they receive the right kind of help. While ADHD cannot be cured, it can be managed. With the right combination of treatments, people with ADHD can thrive at school, at work, and in daily life.

A Combination of Approaches

To be successful, ADHD treatment plans must be tailored to a person's unique needs. Doctors and mental health professionals usually recommend a combination of approaches—including medication, behavioral therapy, and changes in daily habits or lifestyle—to manage ADHD symptoms.

Effective ADHD treatment depends on a person's age and life situation. For example, young children may start with behavioral therapy before trying medication, while some teens and adults might find that a combination of therapy and medication is most effective at reducing symptoms. Adults with ADHD may also benefit from lifestyle changes that help them focus on organizing and managing responsibilities at home and work. Treatment may also change as individuals mature and their life situation changes. Regardless of the combination of treatments a person follows, receiving early treatment can make a significant difference.

ADHD Medications: Balancing Brain Chemicals

One of the most common and effective treatments for ADHD is medication. ADHD is a brain-based condition and often involves an imbalance in certain brain chemicals, especially the neurotransmitters dopamine and norepinephrine. This chemical

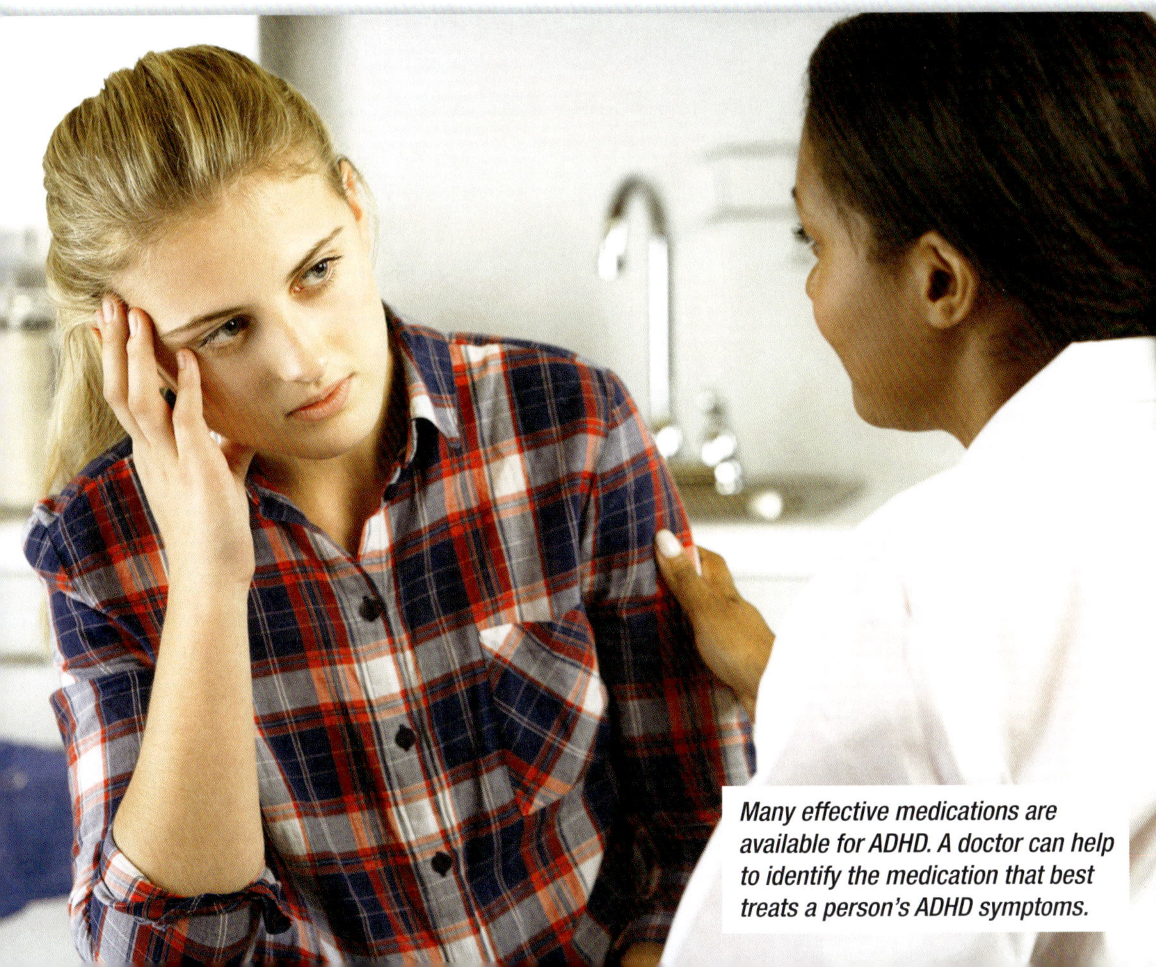

Many effective medications are available for ADHD. A doctor can help to identify the medication that best treats a person's ADHD symptoms.

imbalance affects a person's thinking, motivation, and behavior. Therefore, medication that adjusts the balance of brain chemicals can help a person focus, ignore distractions, pay attention, and control behavior. Medication does not cure ADHD, but it can help manage and ease its symptoms.

ADHD medications fall into two main categories: stimulants and nonstimulants. Stimulants are the most widely used ADHD medications. Stimulant ADHD medications work by increasing the levels of dopamine and norepinephrine in the brain. These neurotransmitters play a crucial role in attention and motivation. Approximately 80 percent of children with ADHD experience fewer symptoms when taking a stimulant medication, according to the Cleveland Clinic.

Stimulant ADHD medications can be short acting, intermediate acting, or long acting, depending on how long they stay active in the body. Some people take them once in the morning, while others may need a second dose later in the day. Most people notice improvements in focus and behavior within thirty to sixty minutes of taking the medication. Stimulants are often the first treatment option for ADHD because they work quickly and effectively for most individuals. Stimulant medications are considered controlled substances because they have the potential to be addictive. As a result, stimulants are often tightly regulated and can only be used under a doctor's supervision.

Social Skills Training

Many children and teens with ADHD struggle with social interactions. They may interrupt others, miss social cues, or struggle with waiting their turn. This can lead to problems with making or keeping friends. Social skills training teaches the basics of how to get along with others. Often conducted in small groups headed by a therapist, social skills training allows participants to role-play different situations, such as starting and ending conversations, taking turns in group games, respecting others' personal space, apologizing, handling disagreements, and actively listening. Within these sessions, therapists provide instruction, model behavior, and offer corrective feedback as patients practice within safe, simulated social situations. Some therapists might also ask patients to do homework by utilizing the skills in encounters outside of class. Learning these skills can help improve relationships at school and in everyday life.

John was first prescribed a stimulant medication to treat ADHD when he was in the eighth grade. The medication helped the teen get through his classes, especially English, in which he struggled to focus. "It would make it so that if I tried to pay attention, I would be able," he says of the medication. "It would still be very boring, but I was able to finish books and pay attention to what was happening."[20]

Some people find that nonstimulant ADHD medication works better for them. They may want to avoid the side effects of stimulants or may have medical reasons that prevent them from using stimulants. Nonstimulant medications work by increasing the amount of norepinephrine in the brain. Nonstimulants take longer to work than stimulants, which means it may take a few weeks of regular use before a person feels the full effects of the medication. However, nonstimulants can be just as helpful at improving ADHD symptoms. In some cases, a doctor may prescribe a combination of stimulant and nonstimulant medications for a patient.

Some patients take medication called antidepressants to manage their ADHD. These drugs, which are typically used to treat mood disorders, work by adjusting the levels of dopamine and norepinephrine in the brain. Some doctors will prescribe antidepressants alone or combined with another ADHD medication.

Medication Side Effects

While many people benefit from ADHD medications, there can be side effects. Common side effects of stimulants include difficulty sleeping, loss of appetite, increased heart rate, stomachaches, headaches, and irritability. Nonstimulant medications can cause drowsiness, dizziness, fatigue, nausea, and low blood pressure. John admits that the medication tends to flatten his mood. "Around my friends, I'm usually the most social, but when I'm on it, it feels like my spark is kind of gone," he says. "I laugh a lot less. I can't think of anything to say. Life is just less fun. It's not

> "Around my friends, I'm usually the most social, but when I'm on [ADHD medication], it feels like my spark is kind of gone. I laugh a lot less. I can't think of anything to say. Life is just less fun. It's not like I'm sad; I'm just not as happy. It flattens things out."[21]
>
> —John, teen taking ADHD medication

like I'm sad; I'm just not as happy. It flattens things out."[21]

Most medication side effects are mild and go away after a few weeks. In some cases, however, they can be more severe or last longer. Patients should work closely with their doctor to monitor the effectiveness of the medication and any side effects they may experience. The doctor can adjust the dosage or medication until the patient finds what works best.

Mixed Results for Academic Achievement

Some ADHD experts warn that although medication can improve children's behavior at school, medication alone may do little to improve academic performance. "It's a puzzle," says F. Xavier Castellanos, a neuroscience researcher at New York University. "There's a real disconnect between the almost awesome effects on behavior and the minimal effects on academic achievement or attainment. What bothers me is that the kids do more seatwork—you can see that they've done more problems—but then when you test them a week or two later, their scores barely budge. Or they don't budge at all. That's the thing that really frustrates me."[22]

A 2022 study published in the *Journal of Consulting and Clinical Psychology* demonstrated this disconnect between medication and academic performance. The study followed children ages seven to twelve at an eight-week summer camp for kids with ADHD. The children participated in classroom learning and traditional camp activities each day. The children were randomly divided into a treatment group that received a daily dose of stimulant medication, while the control group received a placebo. The group that received the stimulant medication worked faster and behaved better than those in the control group. However, there was no difference in learning between the two groups. "Although it has

Supplements and ADHD

Some people have found that nutritional supplements may help manage symptoms of ADHD as part of a broader treatment plan. Supplements do not replace medication or behavioral therapy in the treatment of ADHD, but they can help with managing symptoms. Three of the most promising supplements being studied by researchers are omega-3 fatty acids, iron, and zinc. Omega-3 fatty acids are typically found in fish oil and can help improve attention and reduce hyperactivity and impulsiveness. Iron is an essential part of producing neurotransmitters such as dopamine and has been linked to improving ADHD symptoms. Zinc is another mineral linked to the brain's ability to regulate dopamine and may improve the effectiveness of ADHD medication. More research is needed to better understand the impact of supplements on ADHD symptoms. Before starting any supplement, individuals should consult their doctor to ensure there are no harmful interactions with any medications they are currently taking.

been believed for decades that medication effects on academic seatwork productivity and classroom behavior would translate into improved learning of new academic material, we found no such translation,"[23] the study authors wrote.

Yet many children and teens who take medication for ADHD believe it is essential for their school performance. Martha Farah, a cognitive neuroscientist at the University of Pennsylvania, offers an explanation. Based on her research, subjects who took ADHD medication believe they did better and felt more confident, even if their actual abilities did not significantly improve.

Behavioral Therapy: Building Coping Skills

While medication adjusts the brain chemicals involved in ADHD, behavioral therapy helps people learn to recognize unhelpful behaviors and substitute positive behaviors and habits. Behavioral therapy can help people of all ages manage ADHD symptoms.

For children with ADHD, behavioral therapy is an important part of an effective treatment plan. Children with ADHD can often exhibit disruptive behaviors at school and home, which can impact their school success and relationships with family and friends. Behavioral therapy can help children improve their ability to self-regulate and reduce disruptive behaviors.

For young children with ADHD, behavioral therapy typically begins with parent training. In parent training, families learn how to respond to a child's behavior in ways that encourage positive changes. Parents learn how to set routines and give their child clear instructions. They learn how to use reward systems such as sticker charts to encourage positive behaviors instead of resorting to harsh punishments. Parents also practice remaining calm in different situations and create a supportive environment for their child. These techniques, when used consistently, often help young children with ADHD improve focus, reduce emotional outbursts, and show more positive behaviors.

For older children, teens, and adults, cognitive behavioral therapy (CBT) is an effective form of behavioral therapy. CBT typically occurs in a one-on-one setting with a therapist, but it can also happen as part of a group therapy session. CBT teaches individuals how to recognize negative thoughts and replace them with more positive thoughts and behaviors. In CBT, people learn how

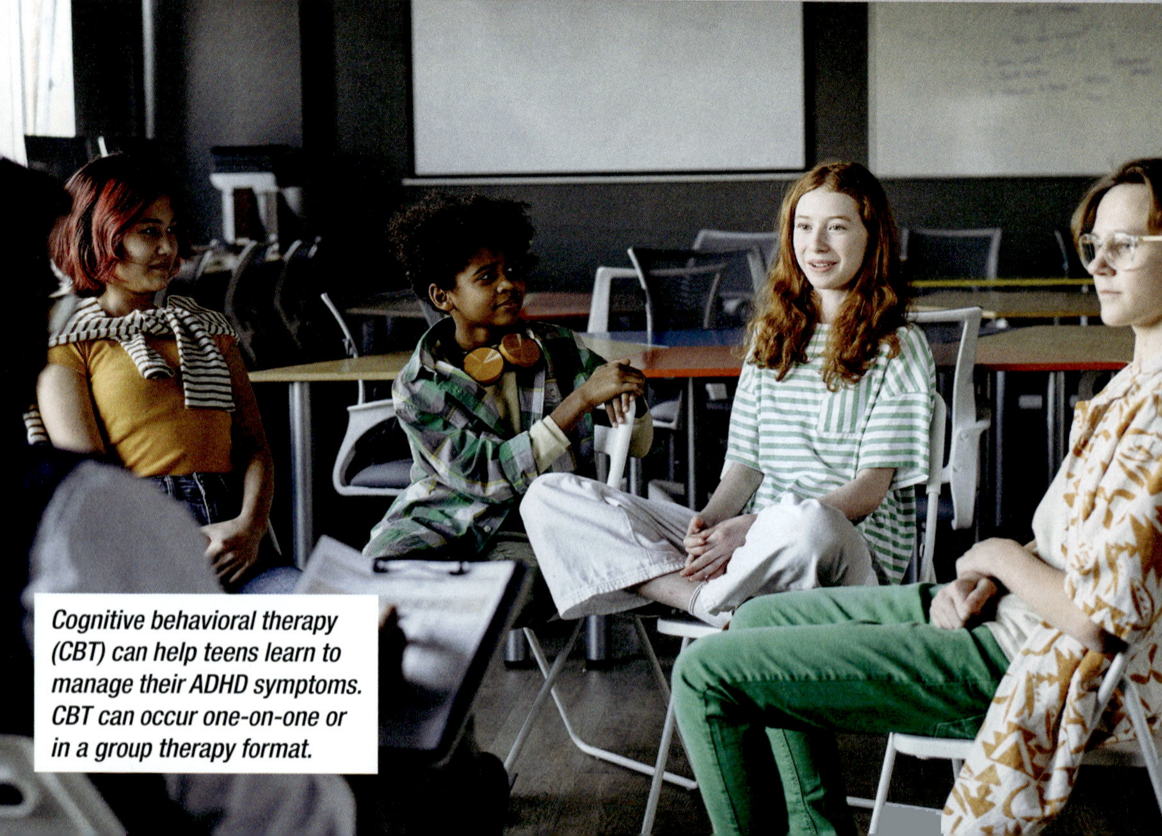

Cognitive behavioral therapy (CBT) can help teens learn to manage their ADHD symptoms. CBT can occur one-on-one or in a group therapy format.

their thoughts affect their actions. They start to recognize negative thoughts and challenge them. CBT can also help individuals develop strategies to improve time management, planning, and organizational skills. They learn how to effectively handle stress and frustration caused by ADHD. Through CBT, individuals build confidence that they can manage ADHD successfully, which improves self-esteem.

Lifestyle Changes: Everyday Habits That Help

Medication and therapy are powerful tools, but daily routines and healthy habits also play a big role in managing ADHD. Making small changes to sleep, nutrition, activity levels, and organization can greatly improve a person's focus, behavior, and mood. One of the most important lifestyle changes is ensuring that a person gets enough sleep. People with ADHD often have trouble sleeping when their minds race or they struggle to settle down. Poor sleep can make problems with inattention, irritability, and impulsiveness worse. Establishing a regular sleep schedule, avoiding screens before bedtime, using calming bedtime routines, and creating a cool, dark, and quiet sleep environment all help improve sleep and give the brain the time it needs to recharge for the next day.

Physical exercise is another way to support brain health and manage ADHD symptoms. Physical activity releases brain chemicals such as dopamine that improve mood and attention. Regular exercise can decrease hyperactivity and restlessness, improve focus and memory, and lower stress and anxiety. Jackson, a twenty-one-year-old living with ADHD, has made exercise a part of his daily routine. "I figured out that, while I'm exercising, I don't have trouble concentrating on anything," he says. Jackson runs almost every day and also does regular resistance training. "When I started exercising, I suddenly was able to concentrate on things that were important to me. There's never been any question in my mind that exercise is related to concentration. Once I made this

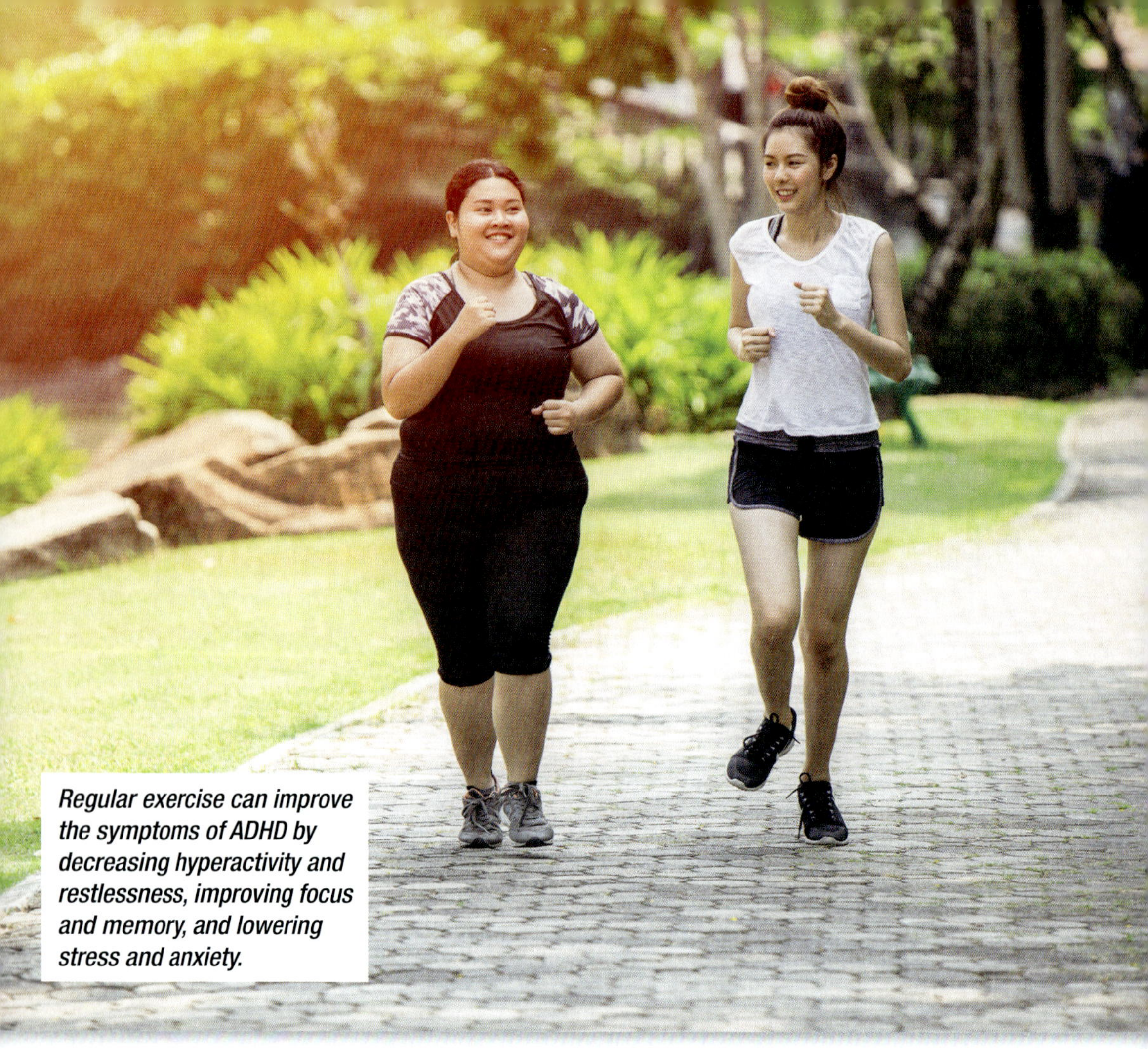

Regular exercise can improve the symptoms of ADHD by decreasing hyperactivity and restlessness, improving focus and memory, and lowering stress and anxiety.

huge life change, and committed to exercise, it was very clear to me that things started to change in my life,"[24] he says.

Nutritious food fuels the brain. Eating a balanced diet helps people with ADHD feel more alert and ready to focus. Skipping meals or eating too much sugar can lead to energy crashes and poor concentration. A healthy ADHD-friendly diet includes whole grains, lean proteins, fruits and vegetables, healthy fats from nuts, seeds, or fish, and plenty of water. Some people find that avoiding artificial food dyes, preservatives, or allergens such as gluten or dairy helps reduce ADHD symptoms.

"I figured out that, while I'm exercising, I don't have trouble concentrating on anything."[24]

—Jackson, young adult with ADHD

Finding the Right Treatment for Success

With the right support, people with ADHD can lead happy, successful, and productive lives. Finding the right combination of treatments takes time, patience, and teamwork. Parents, teachers, doctors, and therapists all play a crucial role in helping children and teens with ADHD achieve success. Whether treatment is medication that helps with focus, therapy that builds new skills, or healthy habits that support the brain, each part of the treatment plan can help people with ADHD reach their goals.

CHAPTER FOUR

ADHD and School

Throughout her school years, seventeen-year-old Makayla Caliendo's ADHD caused her to struggle with focus and concentration. She was easily distracted and often stared out the window instead of paying attention to the teacher. As a result, she fell behind her peers in learning. "ADHD affected my early grades and information retention. I left those early school years with less knowledge than my peers, and that made me feel dumb,"[25] says Makayla.

To help her catch up, Makayla's parents hired private tutors and enrolled her in summer bridge programs at the local school and community college. "The summer bridge programs were especially helpful. Participating in bridge programs led to less stress, as it helped me remember everything over the summer, which normally, I would tend to forget over those three months off. My skills in math and reading comprehension improved during the summer months, helping me to catch up,"[26] says Makayla.

"ADHD affected my early grades and information retention. I left those early school years with less knowledge than my peers, and that made me feel dumb."[25]

—Makayla Caliendo, teen with ADHD

In the sixth grade, Makayla received additional support at school through a 504 plan, which outlined accommodations to help her succeed in class. Makayla's accommodations included sitting in the front of the classroom to reduce distractions, receiving additional time to complete tests and homework as needed, and taking tests in a separate room. Makayla's mother also enrolled her daughter in an after-school program called homework club. There the teen had a quiet place to do her homework and get extra help from teachers.

Over time, Makayla's performance in school began to improve. Now in high school, she is an honors student and is preparing to apply to college. Makayla admits that she still struggles with concentration and organization but has developed strategies that help her in school. She says:

> I make a homework schedule and stick to it and only focus on one subject at a time. I run an essential oil diffuser in my room while I work, and I sometimes take omega-3 fish oil supplements for concentration. I find that a homework buddy or homework club is very helpful in avoiding procrastination and can make studying fun. . . . I keep track of assignments in a calendar planner, referred to as a "reminder binder," and I color code my lecture notes, with commentary in red, potential test questions in green, etc. Most importantly, perhaps, I'm not shy about contacting my teachers through email or during their office hours if I need extra help. These days, I'm finding that I celebrate my successes way more than fixating on my challenges.[27]

ADHD at School

At school, students are often required to sit still for long lessons, manage complicated schedules and assignments, and understand social cues and roles, all of which can be difficult for a person with ADHD. As a result, school can present a special challenge for students of all ages with ADHD. One of the common symptoms of ADHD is hyperactivity, which means having extra physical energy that is hard to control. While some students with ADHD may not seem overly active, others find it very hard to stay still. They might tap their feet, fidget with objects, or frequently get up from their seat. This is especially difficult in classrooms, where sitting quietly is expected. Hyperactivity can make students feel restless or anxious. They may rush through

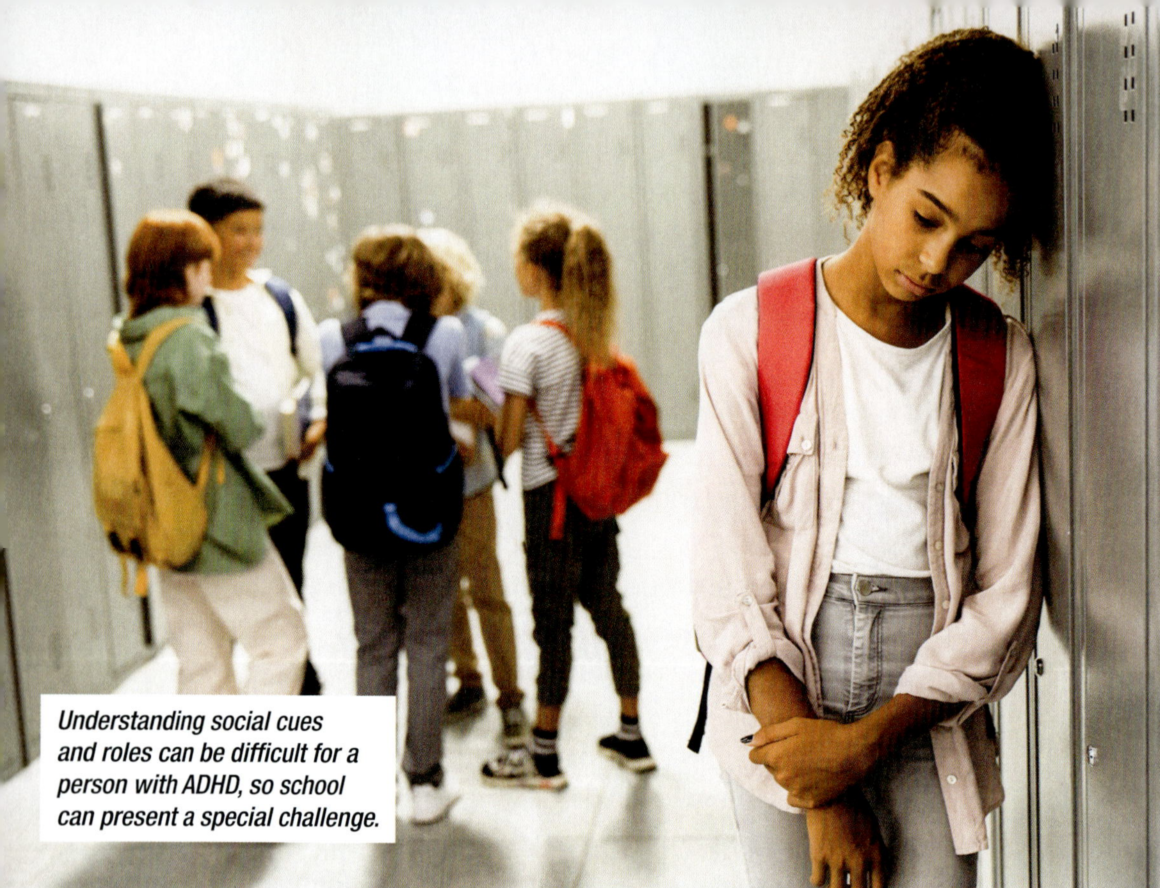

Understanding social cues and roles can be difficult for a person with ADHD, so school can present a special challenge.

their work just to move around, or they may be sent out of class for disrupting others.

Impulsive behavior can also be a problem at school. Students with ADHD often act before they think. They may blurt out answers in class, interrupt others, or speak without raising their hand. This behavior is not meant to be disrespectful, but it is often just difficult for them to hold back their thoughts or reactions. Impulsivity can also affect how students handle their emotions. A minor disagreement can escalate into an angry outburst. Disappointment might cause tears or yelling. This can create tension with teachers and classmates, making the school day feel stressful.

Staying focused during class is another common problem for students with ADHD. Even if they are interested in the subject, their attention can easily drift. A buzzing light, a student whispering, or even their own thoughts can distract them. This makes it easy to miss important instructions or parts of a lesson. Sometimes students with ADHD start a task but quickly forget what they were doing. They may jump from one activity to another or leave questions unanswered on a worksheet. They might read three pages of an assignment but not remember any of the content.

Executive Functioning and School

ADHD often affects executive functioning, mental skills essential for organizing, planning, and managing time effectively. As a result, students with ADHD may struggle in school, especially as they get older and their workload increases. Students with ADHD might forget to bring materials to class; lose worksheets, books, or notes; miss assignment deadlines; or struggle to begin or finish tasks. Without a good system for keeping track of tasks, students with ADHD can quickly fall behind. Even when they understand the content, they may struggle to demonstrate it on tests or homework due to these organizational issues. "Children with ADHD are often bright but lack the executive functioning skills to prioritize and plan, which interferes with getting tasks done," says Roseann Capanna-Hodge, a licensed professional counselor. "The day-to-day grind of endless academic tasks can be hard to manage for a child with ADHD."[28]

"The day-to-day grind of endless academic tasks can be hard to manage for a child with ADHD."[28]

—Roseann Capanna-Hodge, licensed professional counselor

Miya Kofo, a sixteen-year-old high school student with ADHD, understands the impact ADHD can have on executive function and the ability to organize even simple tasks such as turning in homework. Miya often got in trouble with teachers because she forgot to turn in the homework that she had finished. "And it makes, like, you sound like you're lying to the teacher because you're like, I totally forgot this essay at home, and they're like, 'You just didn't do it.' And I'm like, 'No, I swear.' So, now I've come up with a couple of skills to, like, really keep my work together and keep it organized,"[29] she says.

Tutoring and Academic Support

Students with ADHD often benefit from additional academic support outside of regular class hours to help them succeed. One-on-one tutoring can be especially useful, since it allows for personalized attention in subjects where the student may be struggling. Tutors can also help students stay organized, manage their time, and prepare for tests. In addition to individual support, study groups can provide a more engaging way to learn. Studying with peers can boost motivation, improve understanding through discussion, and make learning feel less isolated. Many schools also offer academic supports such as homework help programs, resource rooms, or learning centers where students can go during or after school for extra assistance. These services are often free and led by teachers or trained staff. For some students, simply having a trusted adult or peer to check in with regularly can make a big difference in staying on track and feeling supported in school.

Lower Academic Performance

Because of attention, impulsiveness, and organization issues, students with ADHD may earn grades that do not reflect their actual ability. They may make careless mistakes on homework or tests or forget instructions and miss key details. They might turn in incomplete work or skip assignments entirely. Their performance may be uneven, with better results in classes they enjoy and poorer results in others.

When Meaghan Northup started high school, she received a 50 percent score on her first biology quiz, despite having studied for hours and thinking she had mastered the material. "On the first half of the quiz, I answered every question on biology correctly . . . but I forgot the back,"[30] she says.

Over time, repeated academic difficulties can lead to frustration, increase anxiety, and damage a student's confidence and motivation. Many students with ADHD experience lowered self-esteem after years of challenges in school. They may decide to simply give up, withdraw, or act out in class to mask their feelings. Therefore, ADHD experts stress that it is important for students with ADHD to learn to recognize their strengths and build confidence in their ability to learn.

Social Struggles

School is more than academics. It is also where students form friendships and develop social skills. Children and teens with ADHD may find it harder to make or keep friends because of their impulsive behavior. They might interrupt conversations or say something that sounds rude. Hyperactivity can make it difficult to participate and stay focused during group activities. Emotional outbursts or trouble reading social cues can also make it difficult to form friendships. As a result, some students with ADHD may feel isolated or left out. They may want to connect with others but find it hard to do so in a way that their peers accept.

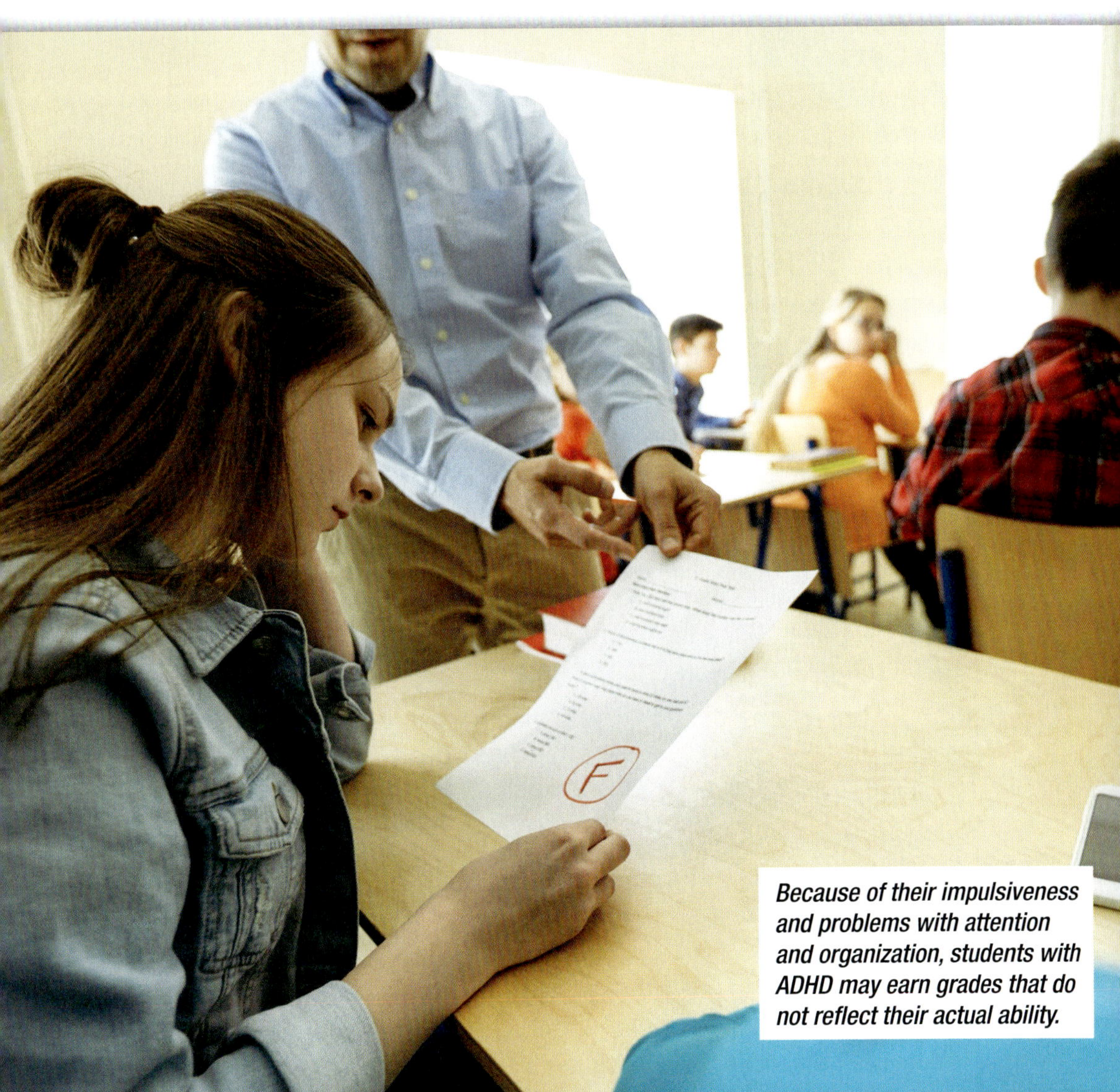

Because of their impulsiveness and problems with attention and organization, students with ADHD may earn grades that do not reflect their actual ability.

Miya Kofo tries to control her impulsiveness and resist the urge to blurt out her first thoughts. She says:

> I've had to really, really learn to think before I speak, because honestly, I think that was a big problem in my relationships when I was younger, that I would just not think before I would speak and I would just blurt everything out. So, now like at least I try. I take like care in what I say to people and like I really think before I say something like how they could interpret that or like how that could possibly hurt someone. And I think that my friendships have lasted longer as a result.[31]

School-Based Interventions

Schools play an important role in supporting students with ADHD. Many students benefit from formal plans that provide specific accommodations to help them succeed, such as a 504 plan or an Individualized Education Program (IEP). A 504 plan is a document that gives students with disabilities, including ADHD, accommodations to the learning environment and focuses on supporting them in the regular classroom. A 504 plan is protected by law and is available in most public schools. A 504 plan for ADHD might include accommodations such as extra time on tests and assignments, breaks during long tasks or lessons, seating near the teacher, help with organization, and the use of technology to take notes or complete work. "Accommodations should fit the needs of each child. Some kids may need extra time to complete tasks, while others might need a different strategy. Teachers and parents can work together to find what works best for the child,"[32] says Ellen Braaten, a psychologist at the Mass General Brigham Health System in Boston.

Students with more significant challenges may obtain an IEP. An IEP is more detailed than a 504 plan. It is a formal plan that includes specialized instruction, supportive services, and measurable goals. An IEP may include services such as special educa-

Daily Report Card

Some schools and teachers use a tool called a daily report card to help students with ADHD stay focused, achieve behavior goals, and improve academic results. A daily report card is a straightforward way to provide students with regular feedback and positive reinforcement throughout the school day. This real-time attention can help students with ADHD stay on track and build confidence. To create a daily report card, teachers and school counselors work with students and parents to set two to four clear, specific goals. Often, these goals relate to the student's behavior, such as staying seated during work time or raising a hand before speaking. During the school day, the teacher tracks the student's progress toward each goal and notes whether the goal was met during each class. At the end of the day, the report card is sent to parents for review and signature. Parents can encourage their children to meet daily goals with praise or small rewards, which reinforces the children's positive behaviors in school. The daily report card's immediate feedback helps students become more aware of their behaviors at school and encourages them to replace negative behaviors with positive ones.

tion classes, tutoring, speech or occupational therapy, or behavior support plans. Teachers, specialists, and families regularly review the IEP's goals to track a student's progress. "Kids with ADHD often struggle not because they can't learn, but because the way they're asked to learn doesn't match how their brain works. Small adjustments can lead to big successes,"[33] says Braaten.

Strategies for School Success

While formal plans are important, many everyday strategies can help students with ADHD succeed in school. These strategies focus on creating routines, improving organization, and developing effective study skills. Routines help make life more predictable and manageable. Students with ADHD often perform better when they follow a consistent daily routine. They establish habits to help with organization, such as using a planner to write down homework, test dates, and deadlines. Visual tools such as calendars, sticky notes, or digital apps can help with time management. These students pack up their backpacks each night before they go to bed. When working on a large project, they break it down into smaller, manageable steps. Many students also find

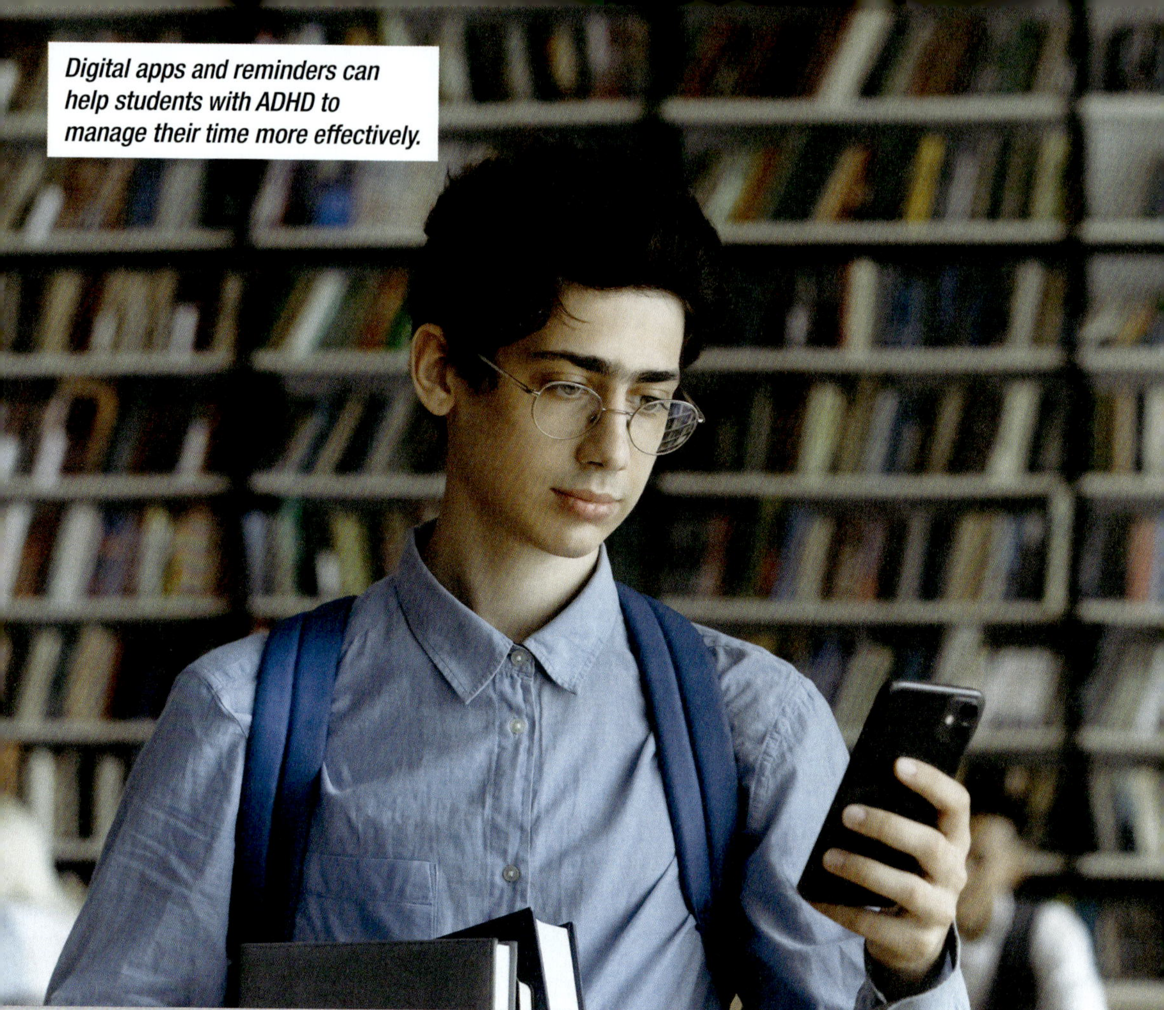

Digital apps and reminders can help students with ADHD to manage their time more effectively.

that creating a quiet, organized space for homework increases their focus and concentration.

Students with ADHD often learn more effectively by following certain habits. Some break up studying into shorter sessions of twenty- to thirty-minute blocks, separated by five-minute break periods. Others use movement to their advantage, such as walking while reviewing flash cards or pacing while quizzing for an upcoming test. Using color-coded notes and diagrams makes learning more visually interesting. What works for one person may not be effective for another. Therefore, students often experiment with different strategies until they find what works best for them.

In class, students can talk to their teachers about classroom adjustments, even if they do not have a formal 504 plan or IEP.

Students may ask to choose a seat that is far from potential distractions to help with focusing. Small tools, such as fidget spinners or timers, can help students focus on tasks and complete them more effectively. Short movement breaks, such as a walk or stretch, can help students refocus on classwork. Teachers can also remind students verbally or with a written checklist to help them stay on track.

Rian Hede, a high school student with ADHD and a nonverbal learning disability, says that working with his teachers has been an important part of his school success. He says:

> Being open with my teachers about my disabilities has been really helpful. They have been very supportive. They've helped me come up with strategies to manage my workload and my learning style. For example, I often struggle with written assignments, so my teachers will allow me to submit audio recordings instead. This helps me communicate my ideas more effectively and reduces my stress levels. I also have extra time on tests and assignments, which allows me to work at my own pace and avoid feeling rushed. I've learned that it's important for me to take breaks throughout the day, like taking a walk outside or doing some deep breathing exercises.[34]

> **"With the right support, kids with ADHD can succeed in school and in life."[35]**
>
> **—Ellen Braaten, psychologist at Mass General Brigham**

ADHD can present challenges in school, but they are not insurmountable. "With the right support, kids with ADHD can succeed in school and in life. When parents and teachers understand how ADHD affects learning and behavior, they can create a plan that works for each child. Simple changes, like making routines, giving accommodations, and staying flexible, can make a big difference. With patience and teamwork, kids with ADHD can face challenges, build confidence, and reach their goals,"[35] says Braaten.

CHAPTER FIVE

Living with ADHD

Michael Phelps is one of the most successful athletes in Olympic history. He has earned twenty-three gold medals in swimming and become a worldwide sports icon. What makes his achievements even more remarkable is that he lives with ADHD. Diagnosed at age nine, Phelps had a hard time controlling his energy and paying attention in school. These struggles made it difficult for him to succeed academically and get along with his peers. He often struggled to stay seated or concentrate on tasks, which resulted in low grades and difficulties with his teachers. "I was told by one of his teachers that he couldn't focus on anything," says his mother, Debbie Phelps. "That just hit my heart. It made me want to prove everyone wrong. I knew that, if I collaborated with Michael, he could achieve anything he set his mind to."[36]

Debbie realized that her son needed a productive way to release his energy, so she encouraged him to start swimming. The sport's structured practices and routines gave Phelps a sense of order and discipline. Regular practice helped him release his energy in a positive way. It took time for Phelps to learn what worked best for him to manage his ADHD. He was often frustrated when he experienced setbacks, especially when his ADHD symptoms got in the way. But Phelps learned how to use strategies to manage his symptoms. He set clear, realistic goals, which kept him on track and helped him stay focused and motivated. He also learned to use mental imagery and visualization to prepare for his races, which reduced anxiety and helped him swim faster.

Over time, Phelps turned his ADHD into an asset in the pool. His high energy levels and sharp focus when competing helped him become one of swimming's greatest champions. And his story illustrates that with the right support and strategies, people with ADHD can live fulfilling lives.

Emotions and Mental Health

ADHD affects more than people's ability to stay focused or organized. It also affects their emotions and mental health. "In the last 15 years or so, we've come to realize that emotion dysregulation is a key component of ADHD," says Paul Rosen, a clinical psychologist and ADHD researcher at Norton Children's Behavioral and Mental Health. "Not all people with ADHD have [emotional] difficulty, but it's very common."[37]

Many people with ADHD feel emotions more strongly than others. They may become frustrated quickly or feel overwhelmed by minor issues. For example, if plans suddenly change, a person with ADHD might react with anger or tears, while others may just shrug it off. This can lead to mood swings, where someone feels happy one minute and very upset the next. People with ADHD might also be more sensitive to criticism, feeling deeply hurt by comments that others might ignore.

These emotional reactions are more than a person being dramatic or overly sensitive. They are part of how the ADHD brain works. The parts of the brain that manage self-control and emotional regulation work differently in people with ADHD, making it harder to manage strong feelings. "Processing emotions starts in the brain. Sometimes the working memory impairments of ADHD allow a momentary emotion to become too strong, flooding the brain with one intense emotion,"[38] says Thomas Brown, a clinical psychologist who specializes in the assessment and treatment of ADHD.

The impact on emotions can also make some people with ADHD more likely to experience mental health concerns such as anxiety or depression. They might feel anxious, worry constantly,

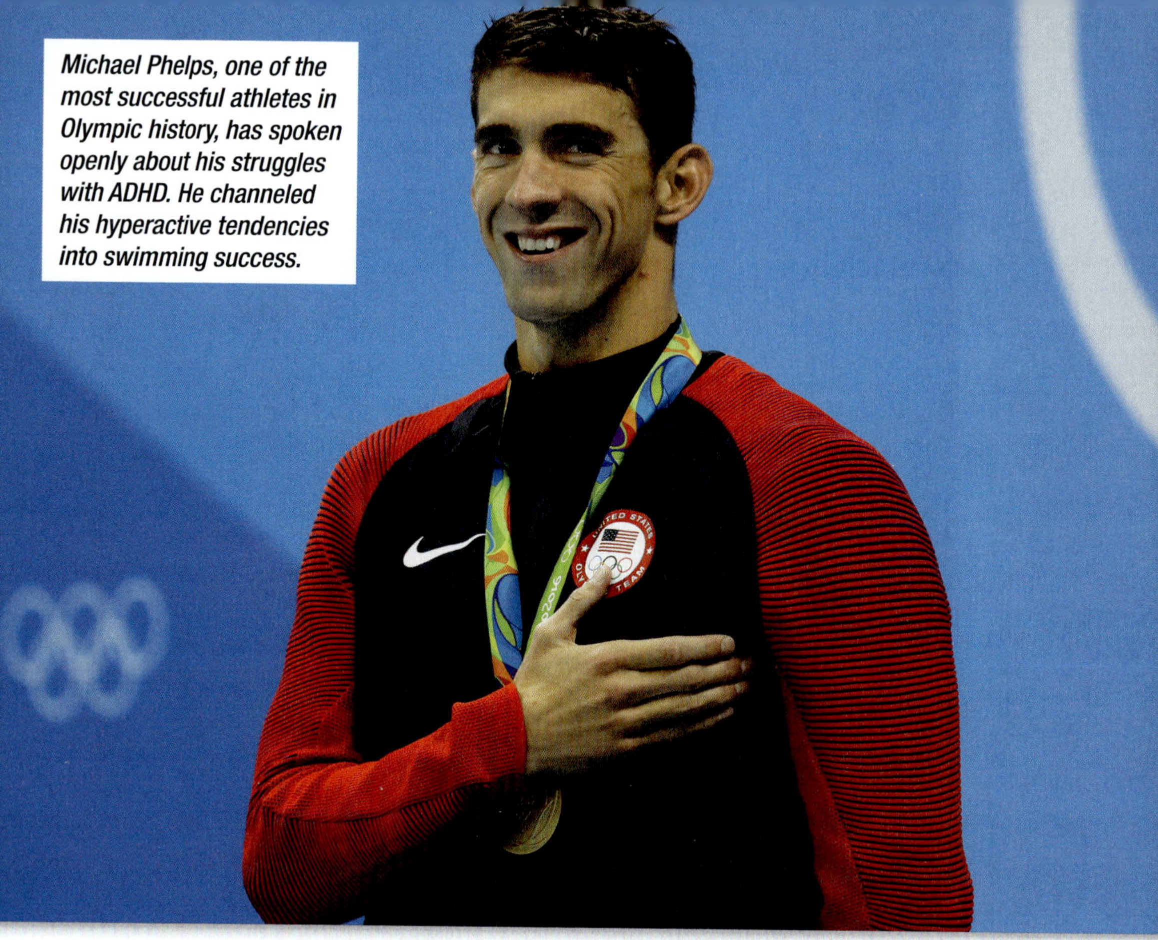
Michael Phelps, one of the most successful athletes in Olympic history, has spoken openly about his struggles with ADHD. He channeled his hyperactive tendencies into swimming success.

have trouble sleeping, or feel scared for no apparent reason. They may feel sad, have low energy, or lose interest in activities they once enjoyed.

However, there are ways to manage emotions and mental health. Existing ADHD therapies—such as cognitive behavioral therapy, social skills training, and parent training—can help lessen emotional symptoms in children and teens with ADHD. Therapies that are specifically designed to focus on emotional dysregulation can help even more, according to Rosen. He created a therapist-led program for children with ADHD to help them understand and manage their feelings. The program begins by teaching children to recognize and understand their emotions. "Kids with ADHD often have difficulty recognizing their own emotions. Partly that's because their emotions can be so strong that they don't recognize more mild emotions. Also, they often avoid their emotions, because they've learned that emotions lead to bad things,"[39] says Rosen. The program teaches participants healthy ways to cope with their emotions and avoid pitfalls such as blaming others, exaggerating, or expecting the worst to happen.

Relationships and Family Life

Having ADHD can make social relationships more difficult. Some people with ADHD find it hard to read social cues or control impulses during conversations. "They miss social cues that other kids learn by osmosis," says Carol Brady, a clinical psychologist from Houston. "Having ADHD is like trying to watch six TV's at once. While you're deciding which one to pay attention to, some subtle information passes you by."[40] People with ADHD might interrupt without meaning to, forget plans, or struggle to follow long conversations. This can lead to misunderstandings with friends or classmates. For example, forgetting a friend's birthday or cutting someone off in the middle of a story might come across as rude, even when it is not meant to be. Over time, this behavior can cause hurt feelings or lead to friendships fading away.

> **"Having ADHD is like trying to watch six TV's at once. While you're deciding which one to pay attention to, some subtle information passes you by."[40]**
>
> —Carol Brady, clinical psychologist

Despite these challenges, people with ADHD can build strong, meaningful relationships. People with ADHD can benefit from learning to recognize body language, tone of voice, and facial expressions to better understand how others are feeling. Social skills classes, role-playing with a trusted adult, or working with a counselor can help develop the social skills that people with ADHD may struggle to use.

For nine-year-old Matthew Bixler, participating in team sports helped him develop his social skills. Before joining local baseball and football teams, Matthew struggled to make friends. "He pushed away every kid who tried to be his friend," says his mother, Stephanie Bixler. "His play was so chaotic that others had a hard time wanting to be around him. He was also greedy with his toys."

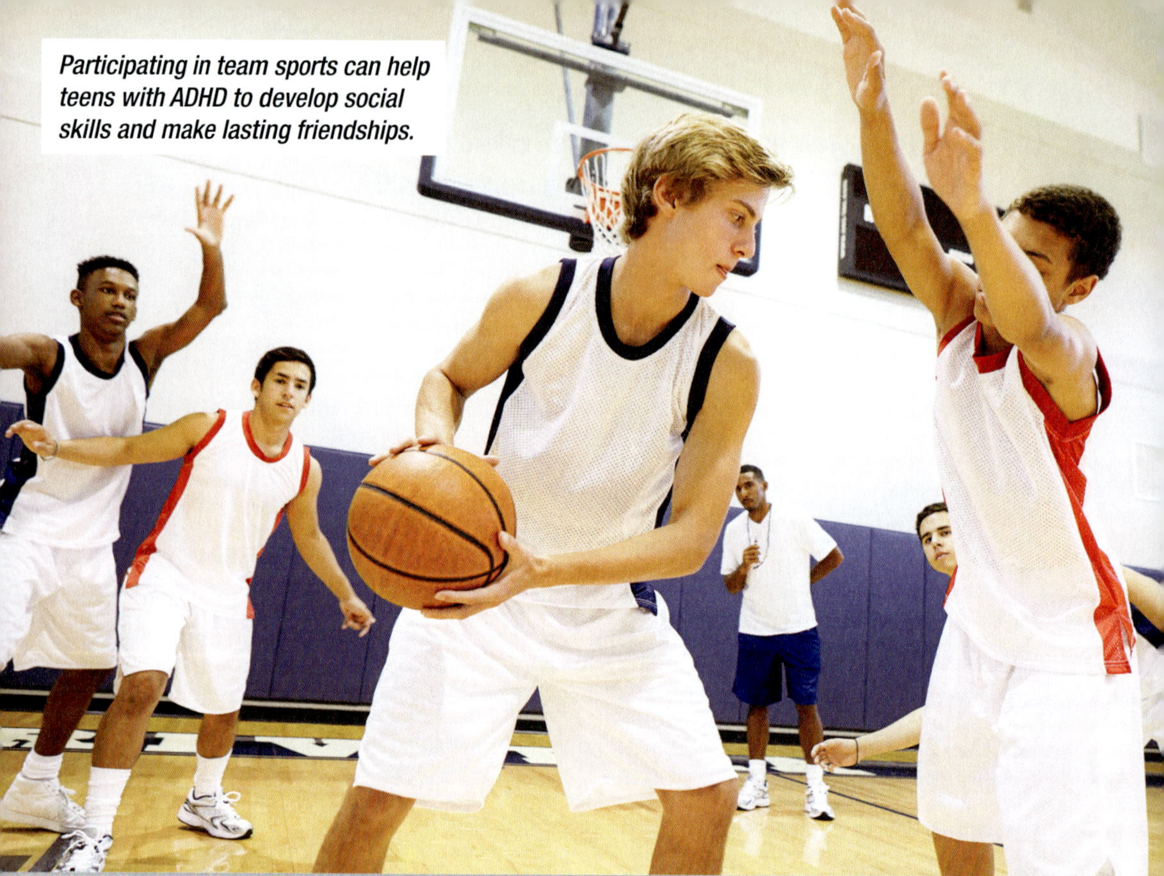
Participating in team sports can help teens with ADHD to develop social skills and make lasting friendships.

Stephanie says that she noticed an improvement in Matthew's social skills from team sports. "He started to realize everything wasn't about him. As the team concept sank in, it overflowed into his play. After two seasons of baseball and two seasons of football, we are now seeing him develop healthy friendships,"[41] she says.

Dealing with Stigma and Stereotypes

One of the hardest parts of living with ADHD is dealing with how others perceive it. Some people still believe that ADHD is not a real disorder or that people with ADHD are just lazy. This type of thinking can make people with ADHD feel ashamed or embarrassed. They might try to hide their struggles or not seek treatment that could help. Some continue to do this even knowing that ADHD is a real medical condition that can be managed with effective treatment.

That is why people like Penn Holderness believe that talking openly about their ADHD can help educate others and fight

> "People look at you like you are broken. But we are not broken, we just have different brains."[42]
>
> —Penn Holderness, YouTube personality living with ADHD

stigma. Holderness is a songwriter, YouTube video producer, and internet personality. He also charmed television viewers when he won the hit reality show *The Amazing Race* with his wife, Kim, in 2022. Holderness uses his platform on YouTube to advocate for those with ADHD and reduce the negative stigma unfairly associated with the condition. He says:

> After I was diagnosed, my doctor gave me a book to read about ADHD that I think got it right. The author said that ADHD is not a *deficit* of attention, but rather an *abundance* of attention without the ability to put it in the right place. He said people treat ADHD like they treat a broken leg or arm. They ask, "What's wrong?" and, "How do we fix it?" rather than, "What is different and how do we adapt?" People look at you like you are broken. But we are not broken, we just have different brains.[42]

Building a Support Network

A support network, a trusted group of people who understand and can offer help, is another essential part of living well with ADHD. Support networks can be a few friends or family members

Tools and Habits for Daily Life

For people with ADHD, daily life can feel overwhelming. But the right tools and habits can make life less stressful and more organized. One of the most effective ways to manage ADHD is by establishing daily routines. Routines help reduce surprises and create a sense of control. For example, waking up, brushing teeth, and eating breakfast in the same order every morning can help start the day smoothly. Following an established routine also helps with managing time, reducing distractions, and improving focus. To be most effective, routines should be simple and realistic. For example, a list of three or four morning tasks is preferable to a lengthy, complicated schedule. Many people with ADHD find that using checklists and calendars is useful for remembering tasks. A to-do list can break big tasks into smaller, more manageable steps. A calendar, either digital or paper, can keep track of appointments, tests, or plans with friends. Technology tools such as reminder apps, timers, or habit trackers can also help people stay on track and make managing daily life easier.

or an established peer support group. "Peer support groups offer a space where you can find understanding, share experiences, and learn from others who are on a similar path. Whether you're an adult with ADHD or a parent of a child with ADHD, engaging with [support] groups . . . can make a significant difference in your life and the lives of those around you," says Suzanne Sophos, a certified peer support specialist who also has ADHD herself. Sophos explains that support groups are not a replacement for medication or therapy, but they have an important role in improving daily life for people with ADHD. "Many individuals find that while medication helps manage ADHD symptoms, the strategies, understanding, and encouragement from peer groups empower them to navigate life more effectively and confidently,"[43] she says.

Mallory Band, an executive function coach, credits her support network, her husband and mother, with helping her manage her ADHD symptoms daily. Band was diagnosed with ADHD as a child and continues to manage symptoms as an adult. Changing routines or receiving negative feedback can be particularly difficult for her and can trigger extreme emotions. When she begins to struggle, Band calls her mother or talks to her husband to get her

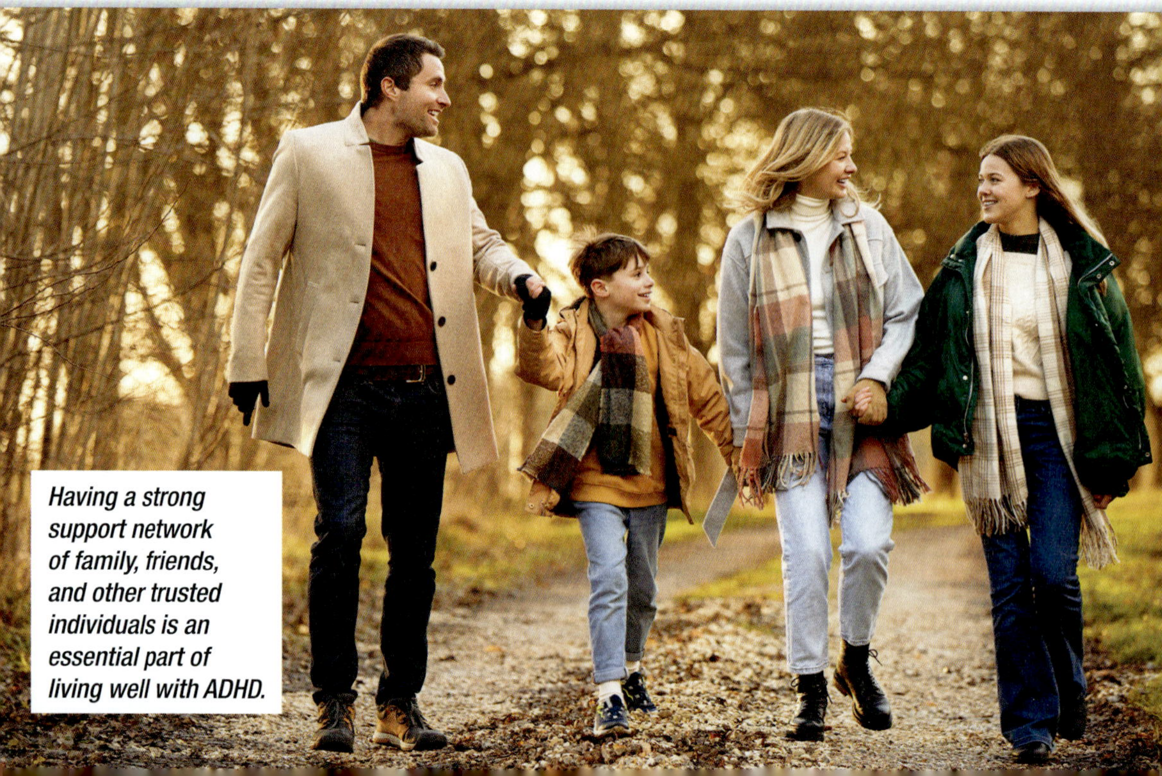

Having a strong support network of family, friends, and other trusted individuals is an essential part of living well with ADHD.

Make It a Game

Some people with ADHD have found that gamification, the process of turning everyday tasks into a game, can help them stay motivated and complete tasks. Gamification turns everyday activities into fun challenges by adding game elements such as rewards and progress tracking. For example, a child might earn points for finishing homework or doing chores, which can later be traded for screen time or a fun activity. Incorporating a timer to complete tasks adds excitement, while visual charts or apps help a person see and track their progress. Gamification can also incorporate social elements, such as collaborating with others or creating a friendly competition, to further enhance motivation. Levels or badges that can be earned through repeated success add to a person's self-esteem and build their sense of accomplishment. By using gamelike rewards, structure, and fun, gamification can be an effective way to support people with ADHD at home and at school.

thoughts and emotions off her chest. By venting to her support network, Band finds that she is better able to collect her thoughts and create a plan of action, which she writes down so she can visually follow it. These steps help Band calm her racing thoughts and emotions, allowing her to manage her daily life. She says:

> Throughout these past few years, I have learned how important and valuable it is to build up a team of support around you. You are so much stronger when you realize that you are not alone, and that you certainly do not have to embark on this journey blindfolded and by yourself. Everyone needs help from time to time, no matter how old or how smart you are. Asking for help is not a weakness, but in fact, an invaluable strength to possess and practice every single day.[44]

Thriving with ADHD

While the challenges of ADHD get a lot of attention, many people with ADHD say the condition gives them unique strengths. People with ADHD are often very creative and come up with innovative ideas and solutions. Many such people are curious and enjoy learning about topics that interest them. People with ADHD are also often energetic, bringing passion and excitement to their

"ADHD is my superpower. I'm successful because of it, not in spite of it."[45]

—Matt Curry, founder of the Hybrid Shop

events and activities. They see patterns and possibilities that others may miss.

Matt Curry, founder of the Hybrid Shop, one of the largest independent auto-repair chains in the Washington, DC, metro area, credits his success to his ADHD. "ADHD is my superpower," Curry says. "I'm successful because of it, not in spite of it." Curry uses several strategies to harness his inner creativity and energy. When his mind races with ideas, he grabs a whiteboard and writes them down. Then he narrows the list to the three most important ones. He breaks down each idea into smaller pieces that help him plan what he wants to do, how he will accomplish it, and why he should do it. Curry also uses exercise and meditation to calm his mind when it becomes too agitated. Curry's advice to others with ADHD is to embrace their strengths and use them to their advantage. "Put yourself in situations where you are going to be successful. . . . Use your strengths to find your own path in life,"[45] he says.

Penn Holderness says that his ADHD helped him and his wife, Kim, win *The Amazing Race*. The couple raced around the world, navigating foreign countries and performing various tasks against other contestants. He says:

> My ADHD was a huge advantage. That was the most comfortable I have ever been. During the show, you can't have any outside contact with anyone. I had one single job with my wife—to get to the end of this race. There was one challenge at a time, and that is what my ADHD brain is good at. I would have been in a lot of trouble if *The Amazing Race* had challenged us to make a four-course meal![46]

Living with ADHD can make difficulties in school, emotional ups and downs, and relationship struggles even more challenging. ADHD may change how someone experiences the world, but there is hope. With the right treatment, tools, and support, people with ADHD can thrive and have full, rewarding lives.

SOURCE NOTES

Introduction: Distracted and Disorganized

1. Quoted in Children's Hospital of Philadelphia, "Attention Deficit-Hyperactivity Disorder: Rohan's Story," June 6, 2022. www.chop.edu.
2. Quoted in Children's Hospital of Philadelphia, "Attention Deficit-Hyperactivity Disorder."
3. Quoted in Children's Hospital of Philadelphia, "Attention Deficit-Hyperactivity Disorder."
4. Quoted in Laura Ours, "ADHD: Misunderstood, Underdiagnosed—and Treatable," *Maryland Today*, October 11, 2024. www.today.umd.edu.

Chapter One: ADHD: A Brain-Based Condition

5. Quoted in Cara Tabachnick et al., "Her Children's ADHD Diagnosis Became the Catalyst for a Mother to Search for Her Own," CBS News, May 28, 2025. www.cbsnews.com.
6. Quoted in National Institutes of Health, "Altered Brain Connections in Youth with ADHD," March 25, 2024. www.nih.gov.
7. Quoted in Sara Berg, "What Doctors Wish Patients Knew About ADHD in Children," American Medical Association, October 11, 2024. www.ama-assn.org.
8. Quoted in Berg, "What Doctors Wish Patients Knew About ADHD in Children."
9. Quoted in Berg, "What Doctors Wish Patients Knew About ADHD in Children."

Chapter Two: Symptoms and Diagnosis

10. Quoted in Australian Psychological Society, "Why Has Everyone Suddenly Got ADHD?," March 9, 2024. https://psychology.org.au.
11. Quoted in Australian Psychological Society, "Why Has Everyone Suddenly Got ADHD?"
12. Quoted in Understood, "Hyperactive Girl, Labeled a Troublemaker," October 26, 2021. www.understood.org.
13. Quoted in Henry Ford Health, "Why ADHD Is Often Underdiagnosed in Women," September 7, 2023. www.henryford.com.
14. Quoted in Henry Ford Health, "Why ADHD Is Often Underdiagnosed in Women."

15. Quoted in Rachel Fairbank, "An ADHD Diagnosis in Adulthood Comes with Challenges and Benefits," American Psychological Association, March 1, 2023. www.apa.org.
16. Quoted in Kara Cuzzone, "The Life-Changing Magic of an Adult ADHD Diagnosis," Wondermind, December 22, 2022. www.wondermind.com.
17. Quoted in PR Newswire, "ADHD Experts Convene to Discuss Appropriate Use of Therapies and Additional Needed Research as MAHA Report Examines 'Overmedication' of Children," CBS 42, May 27, 2025. www.cbs42.com.

Chapter Three: Treatment Options

18. Quoted in Carl Sherman, "Finding Success at School with ADHD: Rory's Story," *ADDitude*, February 17, 2022. www.additudemag.com.
19. Quoted in Sherman, "Finding Success at School with ADHD."
20. Quoted in Paul Tough, "Have We Been Thinking About A.D.H.D. All Wrong?," *New York Times*, April 13, 2025. www.nytimes.com.
21. Quoted in Tough, "Have We Been Thinking About A.D.H.D. All Wrong?"
22. Quoted in Tough, "Have We Been Thinking About A.D.H.D. All Wrong?"
23. Quoted in Tough, "Have We Been Thinking About A.D.H.D. All Wrong?"
24. Quoted in John Ratey, "The ADHD Exercise Solution," *ADDitude*, December 4, 2024. www.additudemag.com.

Chapter Four: ADHD and School

25. Makayla Caliendo, "Pay ADDention™! I'm a Teen Expert on ADD," CHADD, May 24, 2022. https://chadd.org.
26. Caliendo, "Pay ADDention™!"
27. Caliendo, "Pay ADDention™!"
28. Quoted in Sian Ferguson, "8 Ways to Help a Child with ADHD Succeed in School," PsychCentral, June 27, 2022. https://psychcentral.com.
29. Quoted in Understood, "ADHD in Teens, from Friendships to Forgetting Homework (Miya's Story)," September 27, 2022. www.understood.org.
30. Meaghan Northup, "Finding Success at Notre Dame with ADHD," Undergraduate Admissions, University of Notre Dame, September 11, 2023. https://admissions.nd.edu.
31. Quoted in Understood, "ADHD in Teens, from Friendships to Forgetting Homework (Miya's Story)."

32. Ellen Braaten, “Tips to Help Kids with ADHD Focus in School,” Mass General Brigham, January 10, 2025. www.massgeneral brigham.org.
33. Braaten, “Tips to Help Kids with ADHD Focus in School.”
34. Rian Hede, “First Person—How I’m Managing High School While Having ADHD,” CBC Kids News, November 2, 2023. www.cbc.ca.
35. Braaten, “Tips to Help Kids with ADHD Focus in School.”

Chapter Five: Living with ADHD

36. Quoted in Judy Dutton, “Michael Phelps: How ADHD Helped Shape the GOAT Olympic Swimmer,” *ADDitude*, July 31, 2024. www.ad ditudemag.com.
37. Quoted in Kirsten Weir, “Emotional Dysregulation Is Part of ADHD. See How Psychologists Are Helping,” *Monitor on Psychology*, April 1, 2024. www.apa.org.
38. Thomas Brown, “7 Truths About ADHD and Intense Emotions,” *AD-Ditude*, April 8, 2024. www.additudemag.com.
39. Quoted in Weir, “Emotional Dysregulation Is Part of ADHD.”
40. Quoted in Gay Edelman, “ADHD and Making Friends: Helping Kids Build Social Skills,” *ADDitude*, February 17, 2022. www.ad ditudemag.com.
41. Quoted in Edelman, “ADHD and Making Friends.”
42. Quoted in *NIH MedlinePlus Magazine*, “Taking On the Stigma of ADHD,” December 12, 2023. https://magazine.medlineplus.gov.
43. Suzanne Sophos, “Uniting in Understanding: The Role of Peer Support,” CHADD, August 29, 2024. https://chadd.org.
44. Mallory Band, “Providing Perspective Through My ADHD Story,” ADHD Awareness Month, October 28, 2023. www.adhdaware nessmonth.org.
45. Quoted in Eileen Bailey, “Born This Way: Personal Stories of Life with ADHD,” *ADDitude*. April 1, 2024. www.additudemag.com.
46. Quoted in *NIH MedlinePlus Magazine*, “Taking On the Stigma of ADHD.”

ORGANIZATIONS AND WEBSITES

ADHD Coaches Organization
www.adhdcoaches.org
The ADHD Coaches Organization is a worldwide professional membership organization for ADHD coaches. Its website has information about ADHD coaching, listings of local coaches, and information about public events, groups, and classes presented by members.

American Psychological Association
www.apa.org
The American Psychological Association represents professionals who study and treat human behavior. The association's website features information and resources for psychologists, health care workers, and the public about various mental health topics, including ADHD.

Attention Deficit Disorder Association (ADDA)
https://add.org
The ADDA is a global community for adults with ADHD. Its website offers ADHD fact sheets, resources, webinars, virtual support groups, and more.

Centers for Disease Control and Prevention (CDC)
www.cdc.gov
The CDC is the premier public health agency in the United States. Its website includes the latest information about ADHD, including symptoms, diagnosis, treatment, and more.

Children and Adults with Attention-Deficit/Hyperactivity Disorder (CHADD)
https://chadd.org
CHADD is a national nonprofit providing education, advocacy, and support for individuals with ADHD and their families. Its website has the latest information about ADHD designed for parents, teens, adults, educators, and others.

Understood
www.understood.org
Understood is a nonprofit organization supporting people with learning and thinking differences, including ADHD. Its website offers resources for people with ADHD, with a focus on children and teens.

FOR FURTHER RESEARCH

Books

Sarah Boslaugh, *ADHD: Your Questions Answered*. Bloomsbury Academic, 2024.

Amy Farrar and Tabitha Moriarty, *Beyond Distraction: Understanding ADHD*. Twenty-First Century, 2025.

Carol Hand and Melissa R. Dvorsky, *Handling ADHD*. Essential Library, 2022.

Soli Lazarus and Kara McHale, *The ADHD Teen Survival Guide: Your Launchpad to an Amazing Life*. Jessica Kingsley, 2025.

Catherine Mutti-Driscoll and Edward M. Hallowell, *The ADHD Workbook for Teen Girls: Understand Your Neurodivergent Brain, Make the Most of Your Strengths & Build Confidence to Thrive*. Instant Help, 2024.

Internet Sources

Eileen Bailey, "Born This Way: Personal Stories of Life with ADHD," *ADDitude*, April 1, 2024. www.additudemag.com

Kelly Blitz, "3 Productivity Ahas! For Teens with ADHD," *ADDitude*, May 12, 2025. www.additudemag.com.

Shirin Hasan, "ADHD: Tips to Try," KidsHealth, 2022. https://kidshealth.org.

NIH MedlinePlus Magazine, "Understanding ADHD: What You Need to Know," November 14, 2023. https://magazine.medlineplus.gov.

INDEX

Note: Boldface page numbers indicate illustrations.

PICTURE CREDITS

Cover: AnnaStills/Shutterstock

5: Imtmphoto/Shutterstock
9: Pikovit/Shutterstock
12: Roman Zaiets/Shutterstock
15: Kateryna Onyshchuk/Shutterstock
18: VH-studio/Shutterstock
21: Prostock-studio/Shutterstock
23: AYO Production/Shutterstock
27: Monkey Business Images/Shutterstock
32: AnnaStills/Shutterstock
34: Quality Stock Arts/Shutterstock
38: Inside Creative House/Shutterstock
41: Ground Picture/Shutterstock
44: fizkes/Shutterstock
48: Focus Pix/Shutterstock
50: Monkey Business Images/Shutterstock
52: Monkey Business Images/Shutterstock

ABOUT THE AUTHOR

Carla Mooney is the author of many books for young adults and children. She lives in Pittsburgh, Pennsylvania, with her husband and three children.